MY LIFE
FOR
YOUR LIFE

Clarke & Tracie Paris
with an explanation of PTSD
by David Joseph, Ph.D.

MY LIFE FOR YOUR LIFE

Information: www.ThePainBehindTheBadge.com

ISBN: 978-0-615-47288-1

1. Post-Traumatic Stress Disorder—Recognition.

2. Post-Traumatic Stress Disorder—Prevention.

3. Biographies—Police Officers

For information about special discounts for bulk purchases or to purchase additional copies, visit www.ThePainBehindTheBadge. com and select the 'Contact' tab.

Printed in the United States of America

ENDORSEMENTS FOR MY LIFE FOR YOUR LIFE

Read this book. If we will read it, remember it, and apply it, then I have absolutely no doubt that this book will save lives! Our police and military, those who walk out the door every day, ready to trade My Life For Yours... These magnificent warriors deserve the best we have to give, and this book is the very best we have to give on this vital topic.

—Lt. Col. Dave Grossman, U.S. Army (Ret.)
Owner/Director, Killology Research Group

This book is truly a modern-day survival manual written for all present and past peace officers, emergency responders, and military personnel. The contents are founded not only on the author's vast career experiences and current research, but just as important, on the sad and tragic stories of families (survivors) who have personally dealt with the worst side of PTSD and depression; the loss of a loved one due to suicide. The reader will understand how these testimonials, like so many others, could have been avoided, if only the officer or soldier could have been able to simply utter the phrase "help." A required read for students and a must read for all current and retired heroes.

—Sergeant Christian Dobratz (Ret.)
Assistant Professor
Minnesota State University, Mankato

"My Life for Your Life" reveals the emotional pain and suffering that is found in a profession of men and women that bring peace and security each day and night for the 300 plus million people that work and sleep in our country each day. Unfortunately, the cost is much greater to them emotionally and physically than the public may realize. Approximately every 17 hours a Police Officer commits suicide in the United States(Article: "Understanding Police Suicide, author Jean G. Laened, MA. Criminal Investigative Instructor, FBI National Academy, Behavioral Science Unit, "The Forensic Examiner Journal" Volume 19 - Number 3 - Fall 2010, page 64). Approximately, every 58 hours a Police Officer is killed in the Line of Duty. Author Clarke Paris reveals this cultural secret of Police Suicide and what steps are needed to restore the physical and emotional health within Law Enforcement today. John Foster Dulles, Secretary of State in the Eisenhower Administration made this observation, "The measure of success is not whether you have a tough problem to deal with, but whether it is the same problem you had last year." This book provides us answers for today, that will open the door of solutions for all our tomorrows!

—Robert E. Douglas, Jr. Executive Director
National Police Suicide Foundation, Inc.

Law enforcement personnel are routinely confronted with tragic and emotional situations. These encounters impact not only their lives, but the lives of those around them. "My Life For Your Life" is written with the authority of a cop with experience who explains the impact these events have had on his life and how similar events have impacted others. I recommend the reading of this book by every law enforcement officer and their spouse to help them understand that others are experiencing the same feelings and to help them identify when going it alone is not the answer. Paris explains that it's okay to call for backup; in fact, it's the best thing you can do for yourself and your family. This book is a must read through the very last chapter. Excellent!

—Bernie Homme
Former Police Chief

CONTENTS

Foreword by Lt. Col. Dave Grossman, U.S. Army (Ret.)

FOREWORD

You hold in your hand a *lifesaving book* that addresses a vital topic: law enforcement and military suicides.

Every year, several times more cops die *from their own hand* than from traffic accidents and felonious assaults combined. And for several years straight, more soldiers, sailors, airmen, and marines have died from suicide than from enemy action in Iraq and Afghanistan put together.

Research indicates that the police suicide rate may be about the same as the "general population." *But* the general population includes *all* the mentally ill, *all* the clinically depressed, *all* the unemployed, *all* the terminally obese, and *all* the final-stage drug users and cancer sufferers.

For a group of carefully screened, fully employed, and physically healthy individuals to have the same suicide rate as the general population should be a matter of great concern! Every life is precious, and suicide among our defenders, our military and law enforcement, our "*sheepdogs*" is a major threat that we *must* address. And that is what this book is all about.

This book has been written to educate police officers and military personnel, and their leaders and loved ones, on the issues of PTSD, Cumulative Stress, and suicide. And (so very, very importantly) to convince and convict the reader that the psychological help that is in place and immediately available *does work!*

One common trend among these tragic suicides is that they most often did not seek or accept any help. Every cop knows that there is no shame in calling for back-up. Every soldier knows there is no shame in calling for artillery fire. And if there are things happening to your mind and body that you cannot leash in, there is absolutely no shame in getting help!

And my good friend Clarke Paris is uniquely qualified to teach this important and vital lesson. He has "been there" as a "cop's cop" who experienced the depths of depression, who felt the too often unbearable burden of Cumulative Stress, and pulled himself out from the darkness, into the light... with the help of loved ones and the professional psychological support that is out there and available to all.

Clarke is a veteran police officer with 26 years on the job (19 as a sergeant), serving as a Vice/Narcotics Detective, Motorcycle Cop, Bicycle Cop, Field Training Officer and Certified POST Instructor with the Las Vegas Metropolitan Police Department.

He started his "sheepdog" path in the U.S. Navy and moved up to high honors: ultimately to be recognized as the Police Officer of the Year for the state of Nevada and one of the "Most Distinguished Men in Southern Nevada" in 1998.

He has taken his personal experience with depression and suicide to be the creator and producer of the award winning documentary, "The Pain Behind The Badge." He has brought his training seminars on this topic to more than 125 organizations, to include Virginia Tech PD (after 32 students were massacred) and Lakewood, Washington PD (after their 4 officers were murdered in a coffee shop).

Most of all, I would add that Clarke and I have co-trained together, and I have seen for myself that he has the deep and abiding passion that is needed to communicate and contribute in this field. He helps all warriors to understand the vital, lifesaving lessons that: "Heroes can hurt too," that they are not alone with their struggles, and that *"Warriors do ask for help when they need it."*

Read this book. If we will read it, remember it, and apply it, then I have absolutely no doubt that *this book will save lives!* Our police and military , those who walk out the door every day, ready to trade "My Life for Yours"... these magnificent warriors deserve the best we have to give, and this book *is* the very best we have to give on this vital topic.

AUTHOR'S NOTE

"I need help." I couldn't believe the words were actually coming from my lips. In August of 2007 I realized my job as a police officer was beginning to detrimentally impact my life. It was affecting my life in a way I had never expected. The stress was taking over, making me miserable and controlling every part of my life. The stress ultimately reached the point where I had to tell my wife that I needed help, psychological help. This was without a doubt, one of the most difficult times of my life. It didn't make sense; I thoroughly loved my job and never thought police work would be stressful for me. Beyond that, I did not believe in counselors or psychologists. The two things I thought impossible (serious stress from police work and a need for psychological help) struck me right across the jaw that hot August afternoon when I recognized I required help and that help needed to be in the form of a psychological professional.

Once I broke through the wall of machismo attitude and told my wife I was struggling, I began to live again. The decision to tell her I needed help was the best decision of my life. That choice also resulted in the creation and production of my first (and last) feature documentary film, *The Pain Behind The Badge*.

With a lot of help from Jon Giddinge and his company, 100 Watt Productions, we completed the documentary on police stress and suicide. I was confident A&E or another major network would buy the movie. I pictured myself hanging with Stephen Spielberg on weekends and watching football. If you know anything about me, you know it has been a few years since the completion of *The Pain Behind The Badge* and Stephen Spielberg still has no idea who Clarke Paris is.

The movie was complete and I had done all I could to promote the new documentary. *The Pain Behind The Badge* never made it to the living rooms of America. It has, however, been viewed by thousands of police officers across the United States and served as a powerful training tool.

I had begun to feel somewhat frustrated when none of the networks purchased the movie. I had invested all of my money (and some money I didn't have) to make *The Pain Behind The Badge*. When I received a phone call from a police department representative who asked if I gave lectures, I nearly fell off my chair. I was caught off guard by both the phone call and the request, but knowing this could be the beginning of delivering this message to police officers across the nation, I responded, "Why, yes I do." Now I needed to figure out what I would say at those lectures.

That brief conversation was the beginning of The Pain Behind The Badge Training Seminars. It was also the catalyst for this book. As I traveled, I heard first hand stories and learned about officers who had taken their own lives. So many precious lives lost. What an eye opener, and my heart ached with every story. I would picture in my mind, what it would have been like had I taken my own life, or even worse, had one of my children grown up, served as a police officer, and then took their life. Each story was a nightmare and I wanted to do something to help the surviving families and loved ones of those officers. I longed to do something to educate the world on how truly difficult it can be serving as a police officer. I wanted to show officers that they are not alone in being overwhelmed by the stress of their duties. I hoped to persuade them that the help provided for them is effective and that they needed to *accept* that help.

My life for your life, that is what police officers give, not only when killed in the line of duty, but when they commit suicide as well. Police officers see far more than what the rest of society sees. After all, most people won't even see a dead person until a grandparent passes and most adults will never be involved in a physical altercation (fight) in their life, ever. Police officers see and do all of this and much, much more every day. Television has lessened the impact that violence has on our society. It has lessened the impact for everyone but police officers. The violence, hatred, carnage, and death are real for law enforcement. Officers may leave the scene but they take the smells, sounds, memories, and sometimes the emotions, with them forever.

I realize every police suicide may not be caused by the job. However, I promise you that whatever else is going on in a police officer's mind, there are memories of the job floating around among them. You may hear someone say that the police suicide numbers are inaccurate. You might even hear some people allege the police suicide numbers are no different than those in main stream society. When you hear that, I ask you to think of this: A large number of people who commit suicide battled depression their entire life (chronic depression) meaning, they faced an uphill battle from the beginning. Police officers, on the other hand, come from a different segment of the population. They endure a very stringent hiring process to prove they are not especially susceptible to depression. This process includes a background check, a psychological exam and interview, a polygraph, a physical agility test, an oral interview, a medical exam, a written exam, and sometimes even more.

This process is designed to ensure with as much accuracy as possible, that the police officer candidate is compassionate, caring, courageous, intelligent and strong. It is also used to determine whether or not the police officer candidate is psychological stable. All of this is necessary because that man or woman, once they pin a badge on, will have the rights of every person they contact, in the palm of their hand. They will have to make life or death decisions and choices that impact forever the lives of others, in mere seconds.

They will be required to know when to use force and exactly how much force to use. They will sometimes have the weight of the world on their shoulders and America chooses the finest people available for this job. Unfortunately, sometimes the job and all it has to dish out in a weighty moment or over a period of years, is too much for these dedicated men and women to handle—and they ultimately give their life for your life.

The individuals featured in this book were not just cops, they were noble, heroic people who worked in a difficult profession and they are no longer with us. They deserve to be remembered as the heroes they were and for how they lived, rather than how they died.

My Life For Your Life is a tribute to not only the police officers who are no longer with us but a tribute to every police officer in America who deals with battered and molested children, raped women, and all victims of crime.

It is a tribute to those who work graveyard shifts and on holidays to ensure the public's safety. Those who help everyone, even those who call them "Sir" to their face and "Pig" under their breath or behind their back. It is a tribute to the men and women who collectively, are the most impressive and caring group of people I have ever met. It is a tribute to police officers. *Thank you all!*

I want to offer this appreciation to every police officer in America, or the world for that matter. And, I ask that you please realize this truth, should you be struggling right now, *you are not alone!* Please know that the help available to police officers does work. Please take care of yourself. Don't be a statistic. You spend your life helping others. Take the opportunity to help yourself when you need it. Asking for help is not a sign of weakness. On the contrary, it is proof of your inner courage.

CHAPTER 1

COP STEW by Clarke Paris

I graduated from high school in Las Vegas, Nevada in the early eighties. Shortly after I graduated I served in the United States Navy. I have to say that at no time during my training in the navy was anything ever mentioned about stress, in fact, it would still be a long time before I ever had any idea what PTSD stood for or what Cumulative Stress was.

After my relatively stress free time in the peacetime Navy, I was hired by the Las Vegas Metropolitan Police Department. My first four months as a police officer were actually spent at the academy as a Police Recruit. The funny thing about being a young officer, and I have found this to hold true with most new officers, is that I was so proud and excited to be a cop that I wanted to work on my days off—for free. I just loved being a cop. Being a police officer had been my lifelong goal and for some reason I thought that due to my shorter than average height I'd never have a shot at being a cop.

If I were to take you back to the day that I tested to be a police officer, I would tell you of a scared young man standing in the line with approximately thirteen hundred other applicants. Behind him towered two men, both of them probably six feet tall, two hundred pounds with nice hair, (which I didn't have) and they just looked like cops. For some reason, as I looked at them, I knew that I had absolutely no chance of becoming a police officer. I was only 5'-9" tall, 150 pounds, had thinning hair and wasn't absolutely sure what the word "affirmative" even meant. As it turned out, I was wrong. I finished the testing process in the #12 position and began the Las Vegas Metropolitan Police Academy in November 15, 1985.

As I attended the police academy in the mid-eighties, police shows on television reached their peak. "Miami Vice," "Hill Street Blues," and many more drove the image of what a police officer should be. Society thought real police officers were just like what they saw on television. Many officers believed the same. During the seventeen week academy, we were trained in the proper use of firearms, Defensive Tactics, Criminal Law, Department Policy, Patrol Procedures , and on and on and on. There was even a block of training on Police Related Stress. What is so amazingly ironic is that the Police Stress Class seemed to me (and many others) at the time, to be the absolutely least relevant topic for police officers. After all, we were going to be cops. We had all seen the movies and television shows; "Dirty Harry," "Baretta," "Kojak," and "Streets of San Francisco," to name a few, and none of those cops ever seemed to be stressed out. Why did we need to waste training time on police stress?

Until recently, police officers did not dare tell anyone that they were stressed out or struggling with their emotions.

Making any type of statement inferring they were feeling stress or that they could not psychologically handle the job, to a supervisor or anyone else wearing a badge for that matter, was practically career suicide. The saying that comes to mind is "If you can't stand the heat, get out of the kitchen." As unreasonable as that sounds, that is the way it was and that is the way it still is with some agencies today. The tragedy is that the denial of the stress doesn't eliminate it, it merely results in forcing the officer to suppress and internalize it even further, with disastrous results.

Back to the academy... and that class on police stress. I remember the instructor telling a story about being involved in a shooting in the seventies. He was an incredibly dynamic speaker and I remember him becoming emotional as he told the story. He explained how when he was a young officer, he would drive around town just hoping that he would roll up on the Robbery in Progress, see the guy exiting the bank with a ski mask on and a bag of money in one hand and a gun in the other. He dreamt of that. He dreamt of it and knew unequivocally that he was trained and ready and he would "Shoot the suspect without hesitation." He could do that because he was a cop and that was what he was trained to do. He described in detail the avalanche of emotions he experienced when he eventually came across the robber and shot him.

He spoke of looking into the eyes of the man he had shot lying there dying. He explained how he questioned his own actions and that the man he wanted to kill only moments earlier was now dying and he wanted nothing more now than for that man to live.

Before it was done, he was crying. Before he was done, we were all about to cry and we thought "What a powerful story!"

"What an incredible cop!" "I'm glad that will never happen to me!" As moved as we were by his story, I'm positive most of us considered ourselves immune to the same vulnerabilities "I would shoot the guy but I won't struggle with my emotions—I'm stronger than that."

Why did I think that? Why did I think what had happened to him would not happen to me? I thought that because I had been chosen. He had been chosen too, but I guess I thought the emotions he experienced were the exception rather than the rule. I had tested to be a police officer just as did every other person wearing the police badge and just like the others, I answered the question at the Oral Board Interview that was, "What would you do if you respond to a Burglary in Progress and see the suspect exiting through the window with a gun in his hand and he points that gun at you?" Well, the answer for me, as with all of the others, was simple. "I would shoot him." Then they ask, "Would you shoot to wound or shoot to kill?" Anyone who prepares for that interview knows the answer is to shoot for center mass (which means 'to kill'). I never gave it any more thought than that. In that same interview, they asked "What do you think would bother you the most about this job?" As most others answered, my answer was "Children. Children being victimized."

Of course, I never gave that much more thought than that either. I answered the questions, all the while thinking those issues, and others, would not really have that much of an impact on my life. In fact, I pretty much cruised through the first 21 years of my career without a hitch. Twenty-one great years.

Sometimes the Stress Threshold is High

The first 21 years of my career had been flawless. I had received awards. I had worked in specialized units. I had good bosses and bad bosses. I even saw cops struggle just like the academy instructor who told us about his shooting.

Fortunately, my career had gone just exactly as I had predicted when I began the academy in 1985. I had been involved in everything from Officer Involved Shootings to investigating Sexual Assaults, Robbery, Child Abuse and Murder. I had even been run over by a DUI Driver while operating my police motorcycle and my back and leg were broken, but I was fine. I was doing great and loving life. Life was perfect. Perfect up to the end of my twenty first year that is. I really felt as if I had beaten the odds. I wasn't an alcoholic. I didn't beat my spouse. I hadn't ruined my career. Everything was perfect, or so I thought.

Right around the end of my twenty first year I began to notice a change. I noticed a change, not in the job, but a change in me. I started to become overly emotional. The calls that never before bothered me now did. They haunted me with more and more frequency. I had gotten to the point that when I would sit and watch a Disney Movie with my family, I would be the only one getting emotional. It was during one of those movies that I began to realize something was wrong. This wasn't normal but I wasn't going to tell anyone and I certainly wouldn't visit a counselor or psychologist. Something was wrong with me and I didn't know what it was. I had absolutely no idea what was causing these emotions but I knew what was not. It was not my job. I was a good cop and I, unlike so many others I had seen, could handle job related stress. I was utterly certain the problem wasn't caused by my job!

As I suggested earlier, I had been involved in some pretty traumatic events during my career. Each and every one of those incidents were closed by a visit or at least a call from our agency's Police Employee Assistance Program (P.E.A.P.). Each time I was involved in something and P.E.A.P. arrived, I was embarrassed. I was embarrassed because I hadn't killed anyone and my partner wasn't shot. In my mind, there was no need for P.E.A.P. to respond to such "minor" events. There was no need for them because I handled stress just fine, or so I thought...

Two of the high profile incidents that occurred during my career, believe it or not, were not two of the most significant events. The first significantly traumatic event took place at a local bar.

Three armed men entered the bar and began shooting patrons. I didn't get shot. However, eight others did. One of the individuals who was injured was an off-duty officer and he was shot eight times.

Two suspects fled and the other was shot and killed. He died on the ground in front of the bar and one of the off duty officers (my biological brother), and I were the ones who handcuffed him as he lay there, dead. I wasn't shot that evening and I did not shoot anyone. I did however, think that I was going to die. I thought my friends were going to die. It was a violent event and dozens of rounds were fired and as it happened, I was thinking I would never see my family again.

The second high profile event was my on-duty motorcycle accident. While operating my police motorcycle on the Interstate, I was struck from behind by a drunk driver. I was catapulted off the motorcycle and ended up beneath the suspect vehicle. I was transported to the trauma center while, at the same time, the suspect driver was being transported to the Clark County Detention Center to be booked for DUI with accident. The charges would later be upgraded to DUI With Accident Causing Substantial Bodily Harm. I didn't know it at the time, but my back and leg were broken. I ended up having surgery and had pins , screws, plates and rods inserted in my body. I did not return to full duty for nearly one year. Both of these incidents were high profile and could be considered high stress, yet, these were not the incidents that came back to haunt me. In retrospect, maybe it was due in part to P.E.A.P. responding and always being available for anything I needed.

The two incidents just mentioned never seemed to be big factors in my life. They occurred, they were handled, P.E.A.P. was there, it was over. What *did* get to me however, was all of the incidents, events, and calls that most will say are just part of police work. These were the incidents that began to cause the change in my life. The stress. The emotions. The depression. My struggle began, grew, and took my life over and nobody even had any idea. Not even me. My performance appraisals[1,2] for that portion of my career even documented that I was a good cop and I was rated above average in every category... even though I was struggling like never before in my life.

As I progressed through my career, I loved when people told me that I didn't strike them as someone who was a cop, or when they said that I had a great demeanor. That made me feel good. I knew what they meant. I handled stress well and was very proud of my chosen profession. I always told my friends that I would love to climb the highest mountain in the world and shout to everyone that I am a police officer. I don't do that though, because when

I would walk down the mountain to my car in the parking lot, I would find that it had been keyed. Those comments, combined with my police training, prevented me from seeking help once I began struggling internally.

My struggle was easy to conceal. Of course, I didn't realize I had an option. After all, I felt as if anyone knew that things were bothering me, they would perceive me as weak and weak people shouldn't be cops.

I hid these emotions as they came and went, sometimes with no provocation. I buried them, all the while saying to myself that there was no one who could help me and, again, reaffirming the fact it was not my job causing these emotions and not my job causing the struggles.

As my career progressed so did the stress and my emotions, but nobody, and I mean nobody, had any idea of what I was enduring. My emotions would ebb and flow. They were a natural force over which I had no control. I had absolutely no idea what was causing this to happen to me. I did however know what was *not*. It was not caused by my job. The job that I loved. The job of law enforcement. The other thing I knew is that a psychologist or counselor would not be able to help me. I was a cop.

I continued to struggle for several months without telling anyone but I could feel the intensity of my emotions increasing. Then, one day when working patrol, my squad handled several suicides and as a supervisor I was required to respond to each one.

My role in each investigation was minimal but I was required to respond to every suicide crime scene. Two of the suicides resounded loudly with me for some reason; the first involved an 82 year old man who was dying of cancer. The other, the one that broke me, was a 13 year old boy who had been failing Algebra.

Now, I had been on several suicide scenes in my career, possibly 50-100 and many were teenagers but for some reason, this one was getting to me. I recall arriving on scene and observing a man down the road mowing his lawn. I stepped out of my patrol car and walked up to the house where the 13 year old boy lived. As I approached, I was contacted at the front door by the first officer on scene. I then entered the house at which time I heard 10-12 people in the kitchen area and they were moaning, crying, and making sounds like those that might come from wild animals. They were completely distraught. They were the family members of the boy who had just taken his own life.

LAS VEGAS METROPOLITAN POLICE DEPARTMENT
STATEMENT OF PERFORMANCE NARRATIVE
Page 1

Employee's Name		P#:	Review Date:
Paris, Clarke		3082	▮
Rater's Name:			P#:
Lieutenant ▮			▮
Reviewer's Name:			P#:
Captain ▮			▮
	Evaluation Period: From ▮ To ▮		

☐ Doesn't Meet Standards	☐ Meets Standards	☒ Exceeds Standards	☐ Exceptional Performance

NARRATIVE

Sergeant Paris is a senior member of LVMPD. Clarke responsibly delegates tasks to his team members and ensures they are completed on time. He has been pro-active and has developed tactics to address the various spikes and crime trends that have developed in his area. Sergeant Paris understands the importance of setting the example as a "working supervisor" on his team. He gives his team the ability to be pro-active and to take investigations as far as they want, or need. He has worked well to facilitate the development and implementation of positive ideas as well as provide direction for his team, ensuring the right path is followed, and the correct decisions are made.

Sergeant Paris always completes his assigned reports and administrative responsibilities on time. He also ensures that his squad members receive all required training.

Sergeant Paris continually displays exceptional decision making skills and operates within the field environment with minimal supervision.

Sergeant Paris continues to uphold the Departments Fundamental Values. Clarke has clearly demonstrated that he supports the Departments Vision, Mission and Goals. Clarke leads by example, and continues to guide his people appropriately in accordance with the LVMPD Strategic Plan, always preparing for the future.

Rater's Signature:	Date:	Reviewer's Signature:	Date:
▮	▮	▮	▮
Employee's Signature:	Date:	☒ Agree ☐ Disagree ☐ Rebuttal Attached	

(Rev. 12/02) • AUTOMATED

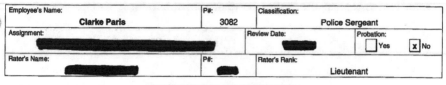

LAS VEGAS METROPOLITAN POLICE DEPARTMENT
STATEMENT OF PERFORMANCE COVER PAGE
PAGE 1

Employee's Name: Clarke Paris	P#: 3082	Classification: Police Sergeant	
Assignment: ▮▮▮▮▮▮		Review Date: ▮▮▮▮	Probation: ☐ Yes ☒ No
Rater's Name: ▮▮▮▮▮	P#: ▮▮	Rater's Rank: Lieutenant	

CLASSIFICATION JOB DESCRIPTION

Foster and promote Department goals by demonstrating Department values; supervise, assign work and motivate employees performing various aspects of law enforcement activities; conduct briefings and/or meet with subordinates to disseminate information; evaluate the performance and competency of subordinates and complete evaluation reports, including praising work of employees when appropriate; investigating, determining and implementing appropriate disciplinary actions; and counseling employees; conduct internal administrative investigations, including documenting, investigating and adjudicating complaints of alleged employee misconduct; identify training needs; arrange for needed training; develop atmosphere conducive to professional growth; develop and/or conduct training which may include academy, in-service, firearms or technical training; monitor and screen calls for service, including observing officers to ensure that safety procedures and practices are followed and hazards reported; conduct inspections of subordinates for personal appearance and maintenance of Department issued equipment; develop subordinate capabilities through goal setting and career counseling; initiate and coordinate Community Oriented Policing philosophies, projects, and tasks; investigate Use of Force incidents and ensure complete documentation in accordance with Department policy and State law; represent the Department at community meetings; give presentations to the public, volunteer groups, and employees related to Department policies or procedures; monitor and control vehicular pursuits, ensuring compliance with Department policy; determine and recommend changes in working conditions, methods, or procedures to improve Department operations; conduct an analysis of current crime trends and formulate an appropriate response; write periodic reports and logs to submit to appropriate persons in a timely manner, including after-action critiques and reports; supervise, conduct and/or assist in overt and covert investigations of crimes and other incidents, including death and accidents; write appropriate reports and declaration of arrests; enforce or direct the enforcement of Federal, State, City and County laws and ordinances; make arrests and issue citations; monitor and review the preparation and execution of all reports and written documents generated by subordinates; organize crowd and traffic control at "unusual occurrences" and/or public gatherings; develop and inspire a service demeanor among subordinates in dealing with the public, including citizens, suspects, and members of law enforcement; supervise and conduct incident actions and tactical operations, including establishing a command post and establishing perimeters at unusual occurrences, and determine need for special units; utilize word processing software and Department e-mail software; stay abreast of current events and issues in law enforcement, including officer safety and liability concerns; perform related duties as required.

ASSIGNMENT SPECIFIC JOB DESCRIPTION

Supervise a squad of Police Officers II and I assigned to the area command; conduct briefings and meet with subordinates reference work performed; evaluate the performance and competency of subordinates and complete performance appraisals; prepare crime information for CMS and make presentations; write tactics related to directed patrol activities and the Department's strategic plan; identify training needs; conduct squad training; monitor and screen calls for service, including observing officers to ensure that safety procedures and practices are followed and hazards reported; initiate and coordinate Community Oriented Policing philosophies, projects and tasks; supervise and conduct incident actions and tactical operations, including establishing a command post and establishing perimeters at unusual occurrences, and determine need for special units; may investigate alleged infractions and/or officer misconduct; monitor radio traffic and code 3 driving; represent the Department at community meetings and give presentations; make arrests and issue citations; write reports and correspondence.

(Rev. 5/03) • AUTOMATED/WP12

After entering the house, I could feel what I eventually termed my pot of Cop Stew, begin to boil. Cop Stew is all of those emotions, fears, memories, and traumatic events that officers deal with, all thrown together in a pot and the flame is on 'high' (The flame may initially be on low, but it seems to always end up on 'high'). I did my job which was merely to confirm the crime scene was secure, witnesses or suspects were located and the appropriate investigative unit was enroute. I also had the ethical or moral duty of explaining to the family what the process was and that counselors would be on scene shortly. Within seconds, I was in a position that I had only experienced one other time in my career.

The mother of the teen was clinging to me, hyper-ventilating, crying and moaning. I had never had anyone squeeze me so tightly other than someone who wanted to hurt me. As I looked at her, all the while trying to maintain my composure, I could see that she was hysterical, hugging me and pressing her head against my chest and snot was getting on my badge and my uniform. I had to get out of there and I needed to do so immediately.

Once out of the house, I made it to my patrol car, started the engine, turned the air on (it was a typical comfortable 115 degree day in Vegas), and then I broke down. I had never cried so hard in my life. I didn't know what was happening to me.

I had responded to teen suicides before and this never happened. In fact, this had never happened to me under any conditions. In the midst of my tears, I heard a knock on the car window. I looked up and saw the man who had been mowing his lawn when I arrived.

He said "Excuse me officer" He then caught himself and looked at me as he said "Are you okay?" He was a good man

CHAPTER 1: COP STEW

and he was genuinely concerned for me. As I sat in the car crying, I had never been so ashamed of myself in my life. He caught me. He caught me at my weakest moment. I thought to myself, "How can I do this job, How can I look people in the eye when they say Thank You or I couldn't do your job." I felt like I had become not only a failure but a coward as well.

When I tell this story to people, one of the first questions I am asked is "Why didn't you ask another sergeant to respond if you knew you were struggling and you could feel your pot beginning to boil?" Because they might think I was a coward (go figure), that's why. Cops don't ask other cops to handle their calls. That was my professional mindset and that is what prevents most cops from seeking help. As for requesting help, I am absolutely positive that had I asked another sergeant to handle the call, he or she would have. It was only in my mind that I thought anyone would think less of me.

This incident was one of the greatest turning points in my entire career. It marked a major transition because after that call, everything in my memory began to return. It was all coming back: dead baby calls, fights, crashes, foot pursuits, rape victims, murder, everything. It all came back and those memories now came back with a vengeance. Calls and incidents that had bothered me 20 years earlier and been "forgotten" came back. As did calls and events from only months before. Some of them were difficult to handle at the time they occurred and others seemed insignificant as I handled them. It was now, for the first time, that I realized my problem was genuinely work related.

Seeking a Solution

You would think now that I realized the problem was work related, I would be able to seek help. Not true. I knew that something was wrong and it was work related but there was no way I was going to tell anyone. I better comprehended the problem, but I was no nearer to a solution.

I had absolutely no intention of seeking professional help either. My favorite statement and a favorite statement of many other officers was "When that psychologist or counselor puts a badge on his chest and a gun on his side, then, and only then, can he tell me how to do my job. This was obviously ignorance on my part and over the next several weeks my life had become unbearable. It seemed as if 90% of my focus was on fooling friends, peers, and family and the remaining 10% was life.

When my children at home would kiss me good night, I felt as if the moment was surreal. It was almost like I was outside of the house looking in as my kids said "Good night Daddy" and then kissed me. I actually watched myself say "Goodnight" back and kiss them. Every day, every evening, every moment had been consumed by all of my returning memories, none of which were good. I had five beautiful children and they were my life. I lived with every breath they took and now my life was becoming an empty shell. A shell empty of all good memories and full of bad ones.

I got up every day (when I didn't call in sick or take a vacation day) and went to work wondering what terrible call was next. I missed my family. I missed them because I was not there emotionally. Depression even began to set in. Now that is something I thought would never happen to me. I was the guy who was always happy, joking, and enjoying life. I drove, I walked, I sat on the couch, and in the yard and I tried to figure out how to fix myself. Professional help would have been the correct answer but as I have already made very clear, I didn't believe in counselors or psychologists. Those quacks were for losers. They don't have a badge, they don't need my co-pay. This is when I decided that the answer to my problem could be found if I would only talk to my wife as I had done so many times in the past.

My wife and I had a great relationship and there was absolutely nothing that we would not talk about. We had even discussed some of the very incidents that were now haunting me. I didn't know how to approach her about the magnitude of my problem nor did I have any idea as to *when* I would approach her.

I only knew that I had accepted that she was my only answer. A couple of weeks passed before what I refer to as 'the day in the pool' occurred.

It was another comfortable 115 degree day in Las Vegas and as I walked out the living room French doors into the backyard.

I saw my wife floating in the pool, listening to music on the radio, and just relaxing. What made this situation even better was the fact my children weren't in the pool with her. Even our dogs were absent which was very rare as they are Yellow Labs and they love to swim. I love my babies and I love when my wife and children are laughing and having fun in the pool but the fact that they weren't anywhere to be seen, made this rare moment my window of opportunity. I knew I had to act and act fast. I put on my bathing suit, grabbed a pumice stone for cleaning the pool tile and hopped in. My wife was so excited that I was joining her that it made me feel bad. She had no idea what was coming her way. This was a great moment for her and a terrible one for me. She always called me her Rock of Gibraltar and now I had to tell her that I wasn't. I was the farthest thing from any man who even resembled the Rock of Gibraltar.

I floated, swam (and scrubbed the tile) for about 45 minutes as I tried to build enough courage to tell her that I was not the man she thought I was. It was all I could do to keep from crying as I scrubbed the tile on the side of the pool opposite my wife.

As I scrubbed I developed a two stage plan. Stage one was to approach her and say, "I have to tell you something" and stage two was to say "I think this job is getting to me." Pretty simple; what could go wrong?

Now keep in mind that for 45 minutes while I worked on building enough courage to even approach my wife, I probably had the guilty look of a two year old child who just soiled his diaper while he was being potty trained.

Once I had developed enough courage, I approached that beautiful, strong, and confident lady floating on the raft and regurgitated the words, "I have to tell you something." Immediately I began crying just like I did the day I sat in my car after handling the teen suicide. You must know that this was not part of my plan, it was completely unexpected.

My wife just stared at me with a concerned and confused look, and kept asking me what was wrong. After a few minutes, I somewhat regained my composure and choked out the words, "I think this job is getting to me." I felt as if a thousand pounds had been lifted off of my shoulders. That feeling only lasted a few seconds though because her response certainly was not what I had expected from my loving, caring, and understanding wife.

I was done. I did it. I told her I needed help. This is where the bad would end and the good would begin. Her response, unfortunately, was not what I had anticipated. First of all, she was neither loving nor supportive. In fact, her response was delivered in a tone that I had heard before only it had never, and I mean never, been used with me. She did not say, "Give me a hug" or, "It will be okay."

There was no sympathy as she responded in a tone of sheer disgust and said, "Are you kidding me?" She was upset and a hug for me was the last thing on her mind. So much for her caress and comforting "We can make it through anything together." My expectations could not have been further off of the mark. She was angry and disgusted with the man she had always considered to be the strength of the family. I didn't know what to do. I knew I had made a huge mistake but I couldn't stop. I began rambling on about dead babies, crashes, fights, fatal accidents, rapes. Everything bad that I dealt with for the past 21 years was coming back, and I couldn't push back the flowing emotions. It was only after I finally regained my composure that I put on my Cop Face and told my wife that I was "okay." "It was just a weak moment," I assured her. I told her everything would be okay and I apologized for what had just happened.

I must make clear the fact that this 'day in the pool' lasted for hours. This was no short event. My wife kept asking me if I was having a breakdown. A breakdown? In my mind, that was confirmation I really was a weak person. A breakdown? Are you kidding me? I cried and my wife cried. It was an absolutely terrible day. It was during the turbulence of all these emotions that I realized I needed help and that, for some crazy reason, I needed to make a documentary movie. (Now keep in mind that I cannot even set my digital watch, and here I was contemplating producing a film.)

When we purchase a new DVD player, we have the company representative install it at our house. People ask, why a documentary movie? I don't know. Maybe I was watching a lot of documentaries at the time. I had never made a movie in my life. Not even a home movie. Despite the awareness of my deep need, I still wasn't open to seeking out professional help. Cop strength (and stubbornness) runs deep.

Once I had made the decision to produce a movie, I began researching the topic of police stress. I learned about Cumulative Stress, Post Traumatic Stress Disorder, and unfortunately, suicide. Even though I had not reached the point of being suicidal, I'm sure I was traveling down that very same road. I just hadn't made it yet to that bleak mile marker. My research revealed some staggering facts. I learned that the Federal Government tracked just about everything *except* police suicide. There was only one organization I could find that had any information on the topic and the numbers they had gleaned were frightening. One a day. One cop a day (including retired officers) committed suicide. That's what the studies said. I took those numbers and ran with them. Now, since the Federal Government doesn't track police suicide, some of the organizations tracking the numbers have their own guidelines for tabulating the numbers. They do all agree that more police officers commit suicide than are killed by assailants. According to the FBI, a police officer is killed approximately every two and a half days in the United States.

When we add together those who perish in the line of duty, with those whose psyche has been so battered and disoriented that they end their own lives, the statistics are staggering.

My wife and I invested everything we had and spent more than a year working on the movie. Thanks to a man named Jon Giddinge and his grass roots production company, 100 Watt Productions, *The Pain Behind The Badge* was completed in March of 2008. *The Pain Behind The Badge* was an official Feature Length Documentary and I naively thought we were going to set the world on fire. Move over "Intervention," "Housewives of Orange County," and "John and Kate plus Eight"... *The Pain Behind The Badge* has arrived!

The film received Best Documentary at the Las Vegas Film Festival and 'Honorable Mention' at the Accolade Film Festival. That is where it ended. The film never received anything more than those two awards. We couldn't be seen on A&E, and we couldn't be seen on TLC or MSNBC.

There was however, a bi-product of the film far more valuable than cash, and that was my health. Filming and producing this movie, talking with numerous counselors and psychologists was my medicine. I was treated by some of the best in the world and it felt great to be well. I was alive again. It was an incredible comfort to know the emotions I had experienced were utterly normal and that other cops throughout the world were struggling with the same issues. I was not alone.

I was however, the fortunate one because I sought help. I lowered my "Cop Wall" and accepted the fact that counselors, psychologists, and every group of individuals who provide psychological help to First Responders don't want to wear the badge—they simply desire to help those of us who do. I now needed to convince thousands of other hurting law enforcement personnel that they too could be fixed. Even more challenging, I needed to help open the eyes of those who were blind to the magma of stresses raging beneath the surface of their lives because they had not yet erupted. Far too many dedicated and courageous law enforcement members are unknowingly sitting on unmonitored volcanoes.

A Change in Direction

I had pretty much given up on ever rubbing elbows with Steven Spielberg and accepted the fact that *The Pain Behind The Badge* was my medicine, and was not a movie destined to be a blockbuster. That was my thought until I received a call from a police agency and the person on the other end of the phone line said, "Do you give lectures?"

There was silence (I think it was me catching my breath from shock) and I gave the impromptu response, "Absolutely, we do give lectures." This was the humble beginning of The Pain Behind The Badge journey of changing lives.

Now there was only one problem. I had to create an entire seminar. Based on the content of the movie, I thought I'd bitten off more than I could chew. After all, I was sure that nobody wanted to hear my story and I certainly couldn't travel and tell the story of other cops' tragedies. Surprisingly enough, it was the common denominator of my 21 year career blended with the careers of other officers that turned out to be interesting to cops. Hearing what I had been through, my struggles, and my cure, was a entertaining and therapeutic to police officers, as well as other First Responders. They were now discovering they were not alone with their unmanageable emotions. I don't think we all need to huddle up and sing "Kumbayah," but without the compassionate personality traits that make these men and women great police officers, they would be nothing more than mindless, heartless robots.

Society does not want robots. They want brave men and women who care about the members of the community they serve. Unfortunately, the seedy side of life, the part that most citizens never see, can take a harsh toll on our nation's first responders. My favorite saying is, "Without fear there can be no courage." I believe that statement wraps up what it means to be a cop, a firefighter, a military member—a hero.

The Pain Behind The Badge Seminar grew in popularity and exposure. As you can imagine, attendees asked what inspired me to produce this documentary movie based on police stress and suicide. Initially I didn't even have the courage to tell the personal story I just wrote about. I would just say that I saw officers struggling and I wanted to help. I wanted to retain some distance and preserve the image I had nurtured over the years that I could handle whatever stresses life dished out to me.

It wasn't until I was speaking with one of the officers featured in the documentary and thanking him for his courage in coming forward to be part of the film, that I realized my not telling the whole truth was cowardly. During the very next seminar I put my heart on my sleeve and told the entire story... including the painful part about "The day in the pool." I was set free that morning and I believe honestly sharing my own vulnerability is one of the key elements that encourages my fellow officers to seek help. After all, cops don't sit in briefings and exchange stories about how they are hurting. Cops fake it. They put on their cop face. They suck it up. They rub dirt on it and get back in the game.

Should they begin to struggle emotionally, quite often they suppress the struggle and fail to handle it in a healthy way. Opting to be viewed as monoliths of self-sufficiency, they end up living miserable lives. And, as research reveals, far too many choose suicide over life.

The Pain Behind The Badge is now more commonly recognized as a Training Seminar designed to help police officers and other First Responders realize that, should they be struggling, they are not alone and that the help in place does work. Our departments and agencies, our law enforcement colleagues, and most importantly our loved ones all want us to accept the help that is available. Our chaplains, peer counselors and psychologists are all trained and eager to stand by our side and help us regain a healthy perspective so we can continue to enjoy a safe successful career.

Let me ask you a simple question. If you knew a fellow officer intended to take his or her own life, would you just stand by and watch? Of course not. You would do everything humanly possible to dissuade them from their fateful choice and save their life. Well, if the day ever arrives when *you* feel there is no alternative but to take your own life, recall this moment and know without doubt that scores of your friends and family will be devastated by your tragic death—and any one of them would give up anything for the opportunity to help you look past this moment of despair to a brighter future. Never believe the lie that no one cares whether you live or die. You may have made mistakes—we all have—but there are still people who love you. And even if the consequences of your mistakes appear insurmountable, believe this truth: there are people who will count it a privilege to help you and to walk beside you in whatever valley of shadows you find before you.

I wrote this book to honor some of our heroes who were not

able to climb out of the deep, dark, cold hole that I escaped from. If more police officers commit suicide than are killed by assailants, how many are struggling down that path right now without us realizing it? *My Life For Your Life* is a book that shows our diverse nation that cops are good people too and not all who die as a result of the unique demands of their job, die in the line of duty. I hope readers will learn a bit about police stress, and gain a greater understanding of what police officers are made of.

This book is dedicated in honor of all of the heroes featured in it, as well as *all those who wear a badge*. It is written in honor of those who remain alive and those precious comrades we have lost. America is a great nation with incredible law enforcement officers. I pray that a time will come when all police officers who might be struggling know it is okay, even courageous, to ask for help.

CHAPTER 2

A DAY IN THE POOL by Tracie Paris

One of the things in life I am most proud of is my husband, the police officer. It is not only the fact that he is a cop that makes me so proud, it is who he is as a person and how well he represents his profession. My husband has been larger than life to me since the day we met. Actually, he is larger than life to our entire family. Clarke Paris, even though he is not exceptionally tall in stature, has taken everything dealt to him in life head on, and won. He served in the military in the early eighties. He has been an undercover officer, a motorcycle cop, a field training officer and much more. Clarke was even Police Officer of the Year for the State of Nevada. He was the epitome of the law enforcement professional. Why would I ever think he was struggling with what his job dealt him?

Clarke and I have always had a great relationship. We make decisions as a team, whether the decision regards our children, finances, our house, domestic situations—everything. We even discussed situations that took place at work. As a 23 year nurse, and someone who worked in the Emergency Room/Trauma Unit and dealt often with First Responders, I never even thought I would miss any emotions my husband might have had, if any, as a result of his job. After all, I was trained to be observant about people's emotional and mental states. Clarke and I both deal with what I thought were similar circumstances and we communicate very well. I never suspected Clarke Paris would be bothered by what he saw and did as a cop. He is my Rock of Gibraltar and I proclaimed that fact to him, and to everyone else.

And yet, despite our excellent communication and my own extensive trauma experience the fact is that *only a police officer knows what a police officer has to deal with 24/7.*

It was August, 2006 when I was enjoying the swimming pool in our back yard. It was a rather hot day but it was perfect from the vantage point of the pool's cool waters. I was lounging on my floating mattress, the music was playing, and neither the kids nor our dogs, two yellow labs (Abbey and Gracie) were in the pool. The solitude was highly unusual. When talking about this day, Clarke always says he didn't know where the kids were. I however, did know.

Cristina was in her room listening to music, Brandon was playing upstairs, and Nick was watching football. It was the perfect and most relaxing Saturday one could imagine and I was enjoying it as much as anyone could. Clarke was working on the yard, I believe he was trimming the shrubs when he stopped and decided to join me in the pool which again, was not normal for him.

Clarke and I have five children, Jessica, Justin, Cristina, Nick, and Brandon (Boo). Even though Justin was in college and

Jessica was an adult, we were always with our kids. When Clarke joined me in the pool that Saturday afternoon, I was in heaven. We never spend time in the pool alone. We usually have at least three kids and those two dogs swimming with us. Clarke joining me in our pool just made a perfect day even better. I could not have purchased a better day... or so I thought. As I floated around the pool listening to the music and enjoying life, Clarke was wading in the pool, scrubbing the alkali with a pumice stone. And he was struggling. Remember, I was so excited to have him there and cleaning it at the same time. Wow! I did not have the slightest idea of the torment with which he was dealing.

Clarke was in emotional turmoil and suffering and I was absolutely ignorant of his pain. We were probably in the pool together for 45 minutes (an eternity for my husband, I'm sure) before Clarke approached me and said "I have to tell you something." He immediately broke down and began crying. He was crying like I had never seen him do before. Now, my husband can be emotional. He can shed a tear when I drag him to a love story or when a baby is born. He also cried at our children's graduation. I wouldn't call him emotionless and I certainly wouldn't call him a sissy. My husband has the perfect hold on his emotions and enjoys life. When I saw him break down like that, my first thought, maybe because I'm a nurse, was that he had gotten some terrible diagnosis like cancer or some similar disease. I know he gets his physical exam for work every year and I instantly concluded he had received some terrible news about his health.

I did not know what to think as my husband was breaking down right in front of me. I was truly frightened. I didn't know what was going on. Once Clarke regained his composure and stopped crying, he said "I think this job is getting to me." And he began crying (bawling) again. I was immediately relieved (because it wasn't cancer) but within a split second I got angry. I was mad at him! We talk about our jobs! I know what he sees at work and he knows what I see. What did he mean by telling me that his job was getting to him? I was furious.

What had he been hiding? Why didn't he ever reveal to me he was struggling? Were we going to lose our house? What about all of our children who still need to go to college? What about the one in college now? What about this beautiful pool I'm floating in? Did I need to work more? Do you want to retire? You can't do that. We won't make enough money to sustain the lifestyle I had become accustomed to! Do you want to see a counselor? Oh yeah, you don't believe in those people. Do you want to transfer to another section within the department? The response I got from Clarke was "I love my job and what I do. I don't want to transfer to another section."

My life flashed before my eyes. My Rock of Gibraltar had crumbled into a pile of rubble, and I was not going to accept it.

The only thing I was focused on was how this unwelcome news would affect my life. What was going to happen to my world? Not once did I stop to think about Clarke and how he was shattered and suffering at that moment. He was a broken man and I couldn't even pause in concern for the beautiful man I had married.

Clarke and I have always fixed everything as a team and you could darn well bet, we were going to fix this little problem. Clarke went on and on. He spoke of calls he had handled 20 years earlier and calls he had been on the week prior. He talked about fights he had been in, shootings, dead babies, murders, rapes, and on and on and on. I never thought those things got to my husband but they did and on this Saturday afternoon, they all came back and as Clarke says "They came back with a vengeance." This conversation was no short talk, in fact it continued for hours. There was some shouting and a lot of crying. Finally, when all seemed to calm down and we had discussed everything imaginable, my husband, protecting me as he always does, calmly and confidently, said "I think I just had a weak moment, I'm okay."

Women are almost always comforted when their partner says "Everything will be okay" and they mean it. When Clarke said these words, I felt good, for about one second. I then realized that the wall he had worked so hard at tearing down to tell me he was struggling, was being rebuilt. When he said those words I knew we had to continue dealing with the issue; regaining our composure and pretending all was well would be a terrible mistake. My husband was still my Rock of Gibraltar and we were going to fix him. I didn't know how, but we really were going to make "everything okay."

The problem was the fact that Clarke, like most police officers and military personnel, refused to talk to a counselor or psychologist. Even though he was absolutely positive the job was the cause of his emotions, he refused to seek professional help. He recognizes today how his stubborn resistance to accepting professional help was a dangerous decision.

What Clarke *did* decide to do was make a documentary movie about police stress. I don't know why he made that decision. He was not a documentary buff and he certainly wasn't a movie maker. Clarke can't even set a digital watch or our VCR. Whenever we buy new equipment for our entertainment center, he has to pay someone to hook it up. I always tell our friends, and our children will agree, when Clarke says something twice, he's going to do it. Clarke had mentioned making a documentary movie several times. Thus, *The Pain Behind The Badge* was born.

I believe one of the driving forces behind Clarke's decision to make a movie developed when he searched the internet and saw that one police officer commits suicide every day. Most officers are familiar with how frequently an officer is killed in the line of duty, but police suicide seems to be a well kept secret.

Unfortunately, the government does not track police suicide, but there are two non-profit organizations that do. These organizations share the common goal of saving the lives of police officers, but since it's challenging to compile the isolated data, they disagree slightly on the numbers.

Even with the disparity in the numbers, we know without questions that more officers commit suicide than are killed by assailants. This is completely unacceptable in my eyes, and that is why Clarke and I started our mission to make a change.

It was only a very short time after our "Day in The Pool" that Clarke began his research and production of *The Pain Behind The Badge.* Clarke sold his sports car, motorcycle and boat to finance the movie, but, I must say, this movie would have never happened had it not been for the financial assistance from a good friend of ours, Dr. William Rifley, and another man who eventually became a very good friend of ours, Jon Giddinge. Jon was the camera man/Director and owned a small company called 100 Watt Productions. Jon's father was a police officer and Jon agreed to make the movie with us. Jon was the one who filmed and did all of the editing and he did a fantastic job. He became a part of our family that entire year, so much so that at the premier of *The Pain Behind The Badge*, Jon's mom thanked me for making him such a part of our family.

Our Healing Process

People often ask, "What made Clarke better?" The movie made him better. As they filmed *The Pain Behind The Badge*, Clarke spoke with counselors and psychologists. He spoke with other officers who were struggling. He learned that what he was experiencing was not uncommon and he discovered that those professionals he was so suspicious of, really could make him better. Ask Clarke and he will tell you that he really thought he was an exception to the rule. He, and I for that matter, had no idea so many officers were struggling. They are besieged by stress and refuse to accept the help. Just knowing he was not alone with his struggles contributed greatly to his recovery.

Clarke and Jon worked on the movie constantly and eventually I seemed to be a big part of *The Pain Behind The Badge*. Even our children were featured in the movie simply because Clarke did not want to exploit any victims or officers. Our son, Justin, was a detective and Jessica was a dead body. Brandon was a victim of a crime and Clarke was a dead body in a car. *The Pain Behind The Badge* had become our life for more than a year. Clarke was confident that, once complete, *The Pain Behind The Badge* would set the television world on fire.

Every television network was sent movie trailers and Clarke sent letters to every talk show host in the world to no avail. Clarke was wrong, America did not really seem to care about his movie nor did they appear very interested in the police suicide statistics.

Eventually, Clarke received his final refusal and it was from the television network, A&E.

Clarke was done. The money was gone. No one seemed to care about the crisis or understand the purpose of his movie. PTSD and Cumulative Stress seemed to be the white elephant in the house of thousands of police officers and nobody wanted to address it. Then the phone rang and it was a representative of a police agency. They didn't want the movie, They wanted Clarke. The man on the other end of the phone asked "Do you give lectures?" The rest is history.

I just want wives, mothers, sons, daughters, siblings, friends, significant others and all of the others who love or care about a police officer, to understand that if you are not a police officer, you will not understand the job of a police officer. Please know however, that the professionals who have trained to deal with these issues are very good, and when given the opportunity, they do an incredible job of helping restore America's heroes, the police officers and military personnel we love.

These men and women spend their lives protecting us and when the time comes that they themselves may need help, it is incumbent upon us to make sure they seek, receive and accept that help. My husband always uses this analogy: "If your loved one had cancer, you would not wait a month, week, or even one day, you would seek help immediately." Well guess what? The professionals are better, far better in fact, at curing PTSD than the professionals are at curing cancer. We just need to convince America's heroes to accept their help. So, don't be afraid to take an active role in getting help for your friend or loved one. You could and will save their life.

Had Clarke not asked for help, I'm afraid he could have taken the path so many of our heroes have taken and he would not be here today. My world, and the world of so many others including friends, family, subordinates, bosses, acquaintances and just people in our community would have been horribly changed forever. I cannot imagine life without Clarke and his children cannot imagine a world without their daddy. We live in a violent world and the only people who protect us from that violence is our police officers and military personnel. They are heroes and deserve to be treated as such.

I encourage every officer or military man or woman who might even "possibly" be struggling, to seek help. It works, and life is too long to not be happy. I love my husband and I am so glad and grateful he remains with me today.

CHAPTER 3

UNDERSTANDING POST TRAUMATIC STRESS DISORDER (PTSD) AND CUMULATIVE STRESS by David Joseph, Ph.D.

Police Officers and Suicide

A debate rages in the psychology research literature about police officers and suicide. One side of the debate suggests police officers are more likely than others to commit suicide. The other side of the debate notes that although there are police officers who do commit suicide, police officers as a whole tend to commit suicide at more or less the same frequency as other professionals of similar age, ethnicity and social class.

It's an interesting discussion, and worthy of more research, but the debate fails to answer a more pressing question: *Do some or any police officers commit suicide because of what they see, do and experience as law enforcement officers?*

The answer of course is a resounding and saddening yes. In her article, "Suicidality among police"[1], Heather Stuart states the facts clearly: "Suicide is the leading cause of death among police officers. Each year in the United States, two or three times more officers die by suicide than are killed in the line of duty and suicide is the fifth leading cause of death among retired police officers." Well-known police researcher John Violanti reported that 23% of a sample of 115 officers in one sample had considered suicide at some point in the past.[2]

The following chapter will share some ideas about how the particularly intense work of a police officer can intrude on his[3] life and his relationships until he feels that suicide is a viable and reasonable solution. Unfortunately, in these few pages, this chapter cannot offer any concrete hard-and-fast answers. It cannot completely explain the behaviors, thoughts and feelings of any one officer. Each is far too complicated and unique for that.

However, this chapter will attempt to offer some insights about suicide, police work, PTSD (posttraumatic stress disorder) and other issues from the perspective of a psychologist who has studied and worked with police officers for some time. Towards the end of the chapter, I will offer some practical suggestions for officers and those who love them to think about and consider.

---

[1] H. Stuart, "Suicidality among police," *Current Opinion in Psychiatry*, 2008; 21:505-9.

[2] John M. Violanti, "Predictors of Police Suicide Ideation," *Suicide & Life Threatening Behavior* 2004; 34:277-83.

[3] According to research on suicide, male police officers are more vulnerable to suicide than female officers, largely because men in general commit suicide at a higher rate than women do. Male officers are also far more common. As a result, I will generally refer to officers as males. However, it is essential to point out that female officers are by no means immune to the stress of police work. On the contrary, female officers have to balance the stress of the job with functioning in a male dominated profession *and* with the roles many of them play as mothers and wives. Female officers (and women in general) are statistically more likely to experience posttraumatic stress disorder (PTSD) and depression than their male counterparts. The contributions women make as police officers, and the stress they incur from their work should not be minimized.

Alone in a Dark World

An example of Good Intentions Gone Awry

Most of us live in a world where we see the good more often than the bad. We believe the world is essentially a fair and just place where love is more powerful than hate, generosity wins out over selfishness and people generally want to do the right thing when given the chance. This worldview is constantly reinforced as we go about our daily business, not in every interaction, but in many of them. In general, we expect those around to treat us with a certain degree of respect, and to deal honestly with us.

The vast majority of our interactions confirm our belief in the basic goodness of others, partly because people are often good, but also because we as human beings have a tendency to see what we expect to see and to filter out information that does not correspond to our existing beliefs. Though we hear stories of murder and mayhem on the evening news, we remind ourselves that while there are bad people in the world who do terrible things, this is not the norm. We lock our doors at night because it's smart to be safe, but we also sleep easily, not expecting an intruder.

This is a comfortable world to live in, and it's the world most of us prefer to wake up to in the morning, but it's not the world that many police officers inhabit.

On the contrary, police officers work and exist in a world where lies are often more prevalent than truths. Where people commonly mislead, cajole, manipulate, deceive and destroy. In this world, police officers see people at their worst, in their most aggressive, shameless and even nonsensical moments. As people outside of law enforcement learn to expect a basic degree of humanity in our relations with others, the police officer learns to anticipate just the opposite. Where a civilian sees two men talking on the street corner, a police officer sees a drug deal. A police officer might be walking his son to football practice, and talking to him about last week's game, but he's keeping one eye on those men at the corner. Where a civilian sees a man and his daughter selling cookies and candies to raise money for her church choir, the police officer wonders about a scam, designed to play on our emotions and manipulate us out of our money.

As one police officer told me recently: "When I came home from a shift, I take off my uniform and store my weapon. I act like a father and a husband, but I never stop being a cop. Not ever."

For many officers, the more they interact with criminal elements, the more strongly their cynical version of the world is reinforced. The more true their suspicions feel and the more vigilant they have to remain to stay protected and to keep their loved ones protected. As one officer near the breaking point told me a few years ago: "When I walk outside, I constantly check for avenues of escape and look around assessing everything. I never want my wife to feel that way. I want her to be happy and enjoy life. I think the world has been ruined for me. I've come to a place where I know the world is beautiful but I also know it sucks, and I know it is as much scum as it is beauty and sunshine... I don't want her to see the ugly side of the world that I see."

Gradually, an officer might find that he spends more and more time dwelling in the squalid world he sees, and less and less time recharging and truly living in the healthy world he is trying to protect. I am not referring here to an officer spending excessive time at work, although this can happen too. I'm referring to a mental state of being constantly on guard, of living behind an emotional wall that separates the officer from any feelings or vulnerabilities that might threaten his ability to be continuously strong and vigilant. Fear, sadness, loss, love, joy—these "soft" feelings find no place in his dark world.

When something particularly traumatic happens on the job, like a shooting, the death of a child or any number of horrifying events, he has no one to turn to for clarity and support. He is wary of opening up to his peers, lest he be considered weak. He believes he cannot turn to his family. He worries they will not understand, and he desires to protect them from the ugliness and pain. Besides, he has invested everything in ensuring that they count on him to be a rock. In a study I conducted with married male police officers who had experienced a critical incident, one officer summed it up this way: "No quitters, no pussies, no crying. There's no crying in law enforcement. For you as a pillar of strength to have a chink in your armor, that's serious man. You question your whole reason for being in it." The same officer continued: "I have to pretend to be strong. It's the same thing at home. You have to be strong. I don't think it would help my kids and my wife if I broke down and became a mental patient and had to quit my job. That wouldn't help them at all."

Just as the officer in our example cannot turn to his families for support, he is also unwilling to let his fellow officers know what's bothering him. He believes that he cannot open up to them for fear they will consider him pathetic and that they will lose trust in him. He struggles to put the situation out of his mind, but finds he cannot.

After emotionally intense situations common to many critical incidents, it's impossible to remain objective about the actions of those involved, including one's own. Officers often begin to question and judge themselves even when their actions were above reproach.

Take for example the death of a child, one of the most difficult events for any officer (or any human being) to deal with. In this example, the officer responds speedily and kills or subdues the assailant responsible. Afterwards though, he invariably agonizes over his actions: "Did I act quickly enough?" "Did I use enough force?" "Did I use too much force?" "Why can't I sleep?" "What is wrong with me?" These are all common questions. In some cases, what begins as a fervent wish for a different outcome, like "I wish I had seen the gun earlier" over time turns into " I should have seen the gun earlier" until in it's final form it simply becomes, "The child's death is my fault." Now that he has blamed himself, he begins to feel worthless and the downward spiral continues spinning with its own gravitational pull. He becomes trapped in a psychological black hole. He tells himself that his family would be better off without him. He feels sad, lonely, guilty, embarrassed, overwhelmed, hurt and angry, but he can tell no one. He can scarcely admit it to himself.[4]

Some officers will do anything (alcohol, drugs, and compulsive behaviors like sex and gambling) to distract themselves and temporarily escape from these feelings because these emotions are so overwhelming that they appear to threaten the officer's ability to be and stay strong.

---

[4]Granted, this is somewhat of an over-simplification, but in a general sense it is a common and dangerous trajectory that officers can and do find themselves in.

These coping behaviors may provide short-term relief, but the damage they do to relationships is catastrophic. Despite the negative consequences of coping in this way, there is a sense among many officers that admitting (even to themselves) feelings of sadness or fear is an unacceptable sign of weakness. They fear that if they acknowledge these feelings, the dam will break and there will be no repairing it. Careers will be lost, lives will be damaged, and officers will feel like they have let themselves and everyone else around them down. One officer I met expressed this concept especially well when he told me that he couldn't allow "anyone to see holes in Superman's cape." So the police officer presses on, alone in his suffering, not realizing that it is his isolation from others and his need to *appear* strong even when he is feeling overwhelmed, that makes him vulnerable to the very worst of options. Temporary escapes only worsen the problem, reinforcing his sensation of being trapped, helpless and without any options—save one. Over time, a greater and greater distance grows between him and others, until eventually he feels as if he is standing all alone in the dark, lost and disconnected from the people he loves. Having sacrificed all to maintain a façade of invulnerability, he has severed all of the bonds that could actually rescue him.

What to Watch Out For
What the Research Says About Suicide

One of the most heartbreaking aspects of many suicides is that the family and friends of the person who took their own life often had no idea what was happening to their loved one until it was too late. The people who would have helped could not, simply because they did not know how. The following paragraphs offer some specific guidance from the research literature about common risk factors for suicide in police officers.[5]

---

[5]Unfortunately, some people who commit suicide are masters at hiding their feelings. They mask their suffering so well that even the most well-informed, observant family member might not recognize a potential disaster looming.

Depression

One of the most commonly cited risks for suicide and suicidal thoughts is depression. Depression is a mental illness that is often used in everyday speech to mean "feeling down" or "being in a funk," but in reality depression is far more serious than a passing case of the blues. Depression can affect thoughts, behavior and mood. It can cloud judgment, reduce concentration and impair memory. Without treatment, depression can last for weeks, months or years. Depression increases the chances of risky behaviors such as substance use, and can wreak havoc on careers and relationships. Of the many symptoms of depression, the most debilitating two for many are (1) a complete and inescapable sense of hopelessness and (2) an overpowering sense of worthlessness. One officer described it to me as "living in a dark cloud where no light can enter." Some (not all) of the signs of depression include fatigue, significant changes in weight (up or down) and sleep patterns (more or less). In police officers who are not comfortable sharing their feelings with others, signs of depression may not be so easy to recognize. Men tend to express depression through anger, irritability and impatience. Relatively small daily stressors that often barely provoke a response, like a broken glass in the sink or an unpaid bill, might be met with a tirade of anger from even the most even-tempered person.

These behaviors tend to push people away at precisely the time when help is most needed. There are many reasons why someone might become clinically depressed.

Some reasons may be job related, while others are not. Researchers believe genetics may play a role. The good news is that there are excellent treatments available for depression that do not cost a fortune and may permanently resolve the problem in a matter of months.

Substance Use

Drinking and substance use can seem a very effective *temporary* way to cope with the stress of police work and the everyday problems of home, relationships and money. It can aid sleep and manage overwhelming feelings—*in the short term*. If it wasn't so effective, people wouldn't do it! Of course, substance and alcohol use is also the cause of an untold amount of turmoil and destruction for those who use or drink, and their loved ones often bear the brunt of the pain. Substance and alcohol use is also very highly associated with acts of suicide. One of the reasons for this is that substance use impairs judgment and increases impulsivity and for many, the physical act of committing suicide is already very impulsive behavior. One officer related: "I just found myself with my gun in my hand. I don't remember getting it or even making the decision to use it. I had a drink in one hand and my weapon in the other, and all I could think about was how peaceful it would be to have it all over with, and to just check out. I had convinced myself—and now I can see how my thoughts were clouded by the alcohol—that everyone would be better off without me."

To some degree, Hollywood has glorified the image of the tough cop, downing some shots after a hard day of cleaning up the dirt on society's mean streets. The cops in these shows are presented as heroes, tough guys who do things their way. These clichés have little to do with life in the real world, but they may exert some influence over what is deemed as acceptable behavior in certain police cultures. A number of police officers have told me openly and without concern, that they cope with traumatic events by heading to the bar. Drinking (or drug use) is never a safe way to cope, and cops who manage their feelings by drinking or using, often end up divorced, in trouble at work and isolated from their friends. An officer I spoke to recently recounted how he transformed from a rising star in his department and a happily married man into a homeless, divorced ex-cop contemplating suicide *in less than a year* because he was relying on substance use to manage his fears and burnout after years of working undercover.

Access to Guns

It is a little known fact that women *attempt* suicide more often than men, while men actually *commit* suicide more frequently than women. One of the reasons for this—and a very relevant concern to police officers—is access to guns. Men (90% of police officers are men) are more likely to use lethal means in a suicide attempt than women are, so the availability of firearms is a very significant risk factor. Most (not all) people commit suicide in simple ways using means that are readily accessible to them (like guns or prescribed pills). They do not devise intricate plans. Like the officer in the previous example, familiarity with handguns increases the risk that an officer might reach for one in a moment of impulsivity or hopelessness.

Ironically, many officers keep weapons at home to protect themselves and their families from threats, when in fact it is the presence of the weapon itself that can be the greater danger.

PTSD

The symptoms of posttraumatic stress disorder (PTSD), include hyper-vigilance, avoidance (of disturbing thoughts and feelings and reminders of trauma), and re-experiencing the trauma in the form of flashbacks or nightmares. They intensify the feeling of being engulfed by a world of hurt, pain and anger. PTSD, like alcohol and depression, tends to increase the distance between officers and those who could help. Considering the number of traumatic events officers routinely experience (most studies estimate that over 70% of police officers experience job related trauma), the rates for PTSD in police officers are surprisingly low. Still, at 9% they are appreciably higher than those of the general population (about 4.5%). A number of studies have indicated that officers with PTSD think about suicide significantly more frequently than officers without PTSD. Like depression and most other mental health disorders, it is impossible to predict who will get PTSD as a consequence of a particular event and who will not. Unfortunately, many officers associate PTSD with a lack of mental toughness. Nothing could be further from the truth. Just like their military counterparts, some of the toughest, most highly-skilled, and best trained law enforcement officers get PTSD.

One way of understanding PTSD is to see it as the brain working in overdrive. Instead of processing an experience like a normal memory, even a bad one, the PTSD brain does not allow it to settle. For example, in the days following a minor fender-bender, most of us will find that we are more vigilant and jumpy when we drive. We check our mirrors more often than needed, and are relieved when we get to where we are going. This is our brain's way of saying "Be aware! Don't let this happen again!" Over the course of a few days or weeks though, most of us return to driving normally, which is to say we return to driving without thinking of the accident.

In the case of PTSD, the brain does not allow the event to become a normal memory, recalled at will. Instead, the memory and emotions that accompany the memory (like fear and helplessness) are always utmost in the mind no matter how hard a person tries not to think about it. Even when the event seems to be settled, a reminder or trigger will bring it back as fresh as if it was happening again right now. Sleeping hours are invaded by nightmares. Many officers with PTSD complain of getting only 2-3 hours of sleep a night, sometimes for years. The sleep loss alone causes impaired judgment and concentration, irritable moods and difficulty in maintaining relationships. When the other symptoms are factored in, PTSD can be a tremendously difficult and debilitating condition. To make matters worse, it is very common for officers with PTSD to experience either or both depression and substance use.

PTSD and substance use are a particularly formidable combination because they destructively reinforce one another. For example:

> An officer with PTSD finds he cannot sleep because of an overwhelming event that happened last month. In fact, this event is so upsetting to him that he will try to avoid thinking about it at all costs (another symptom of PTSD). He finds that drinking five or six shots of vodka will push the thoughts away temporarily and allow him to briefly sleep. Because drinking seems to work, this is the method of coping that he relies on more and more often, even when the negative consequences of his drinking become apparent to him. Because the alcohol prevents him from really facing and processing the event (the usual therapy for PTSD), or even seeking any help for it, his PTSD symptoms do not improve. Months later, the walls are caving in around him—his job, his relationships are all threatened—and the only way he knows how to cope is making things even worse.

As is the case for depression, there are excellent therapies for PTSD that do not take forever to complete and often help people tremendously. (EMDR, eye movement desensitization and reprocessing, is one popular therapy, but there are others.) While reaching out for help can involve some risk—some departments are more understanding than others—not getting help constitutes the far greater risk.

Feeling Trapped by a False Choice

On some occasions, healing from PTSD, depression and substance use can only be fully realized when the officer changes careers. Like football players with too many concussions, sometimes it's essential to know when to step away. For many officers, the potential loss of a career makes it particularly difficult to acknowledge a problem. Like the officer in the beginning of this chapter who never stops being a cop, many officers have told me that being a police officer is more than a career to them, it is an identity.

To give up on being a cop seems like surrendering who they are. Yet, continuing as a police officer with all of the above happening, feels impossible too. It is this sense of being trapped that causes some people to turn to the one counterfeit escape that seems possible. This is the false all-or-nothing choice of suicide. It is in these instances though, that it is crucial to remember that identities are never singular. We all have multiple roles in life. As one identity is phased out (being a cop) others can be strengthened (being a father, a husband) and dynamic new identities can be forged. There are always multiple paths to healing, and there is always more than one choice. And virtually any choice is preferable to the illusion that suicide is an answer to one's problems.

CHAPTER 4
OUR HEROES

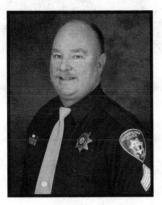

REAGAN ALEXANDER
December 3, 1958—April 12, 2010

Biography by Dawn Alexander (Wife)

Reagan Alexander was a man who had an uncanny ability to make everyone around him laugh. He was an understanding, compassionate, intelligent and strong man of God who loved life and enjoyed its challenges.

Reagan was born on the 3rd of December in 1958 at Lynwood hospital in Lynwood, California to Jim and Ty Alexander. Keith was Reagan's only sibling and was his younger brother. Reagan was raised in Southern California and Las Vegas, Nevada. As a young child, Reagan showed his creative prowess in many ways. He was animated and outgoing; he was the friend everyone went to when they were facing struggles of their own. Reagan loved sports and as a youth he played football and baseball, however, weightlifting was his favorite class in high school.

Childhood was not really much different for Reagan than it is for most growing boys. He had great friendships. He loved action, playing, laughing, and like most young boys in Southern Nevada, he loved to hunt for lizards. Reagan carried his life-loving attitude throughout every year of his life and shared all he had with his friends and family.

The Western High School graduating class of 1977 was Reagan's class. High school played a large role in Reagan's life as it does for most teen age boys. He played football for the Western Warriors and continued to love watching football with friends throughout the following years. Some of Reagan's good friends were Bruce Eubank, Mark Pence, and Al Crissman. Later in life, Reagan cultivated very close relationships with Sydney and Russell Bridges and Sandy and Manual Gonzalez.

The way he always treated people with respect and dignity combined with the fact he was one of the most compassionate men on earth is most likely what attracted Dawn Marie Lewis to Reagan. (His overpowering sense of humor also helped.) Dawn and Reagan knew they were right for each other and history proved their belief to be correct. Dawn and Reagan exchanged wedding vows at the Las Vegas Courthouse on June 16, 1982 in Las Vegas, Nevada. As a hard worker with drive and determination, an engaging personality, and a sense of humor that makes millionaires of some, Reagan was the man whom Dawn knew she would love for eternity.

Some people are good with kids but Reagan was amazing with them. He understood how they thought, what they thought, why they thought, and why they were here. Reagan knew children were the future of our world and if we give to them today, they will give to us (the world) tomorrow. This was proven when he and Dawn were blessed with their three children, two sons, Nathanael and Caleb, and one daughter, Brandi.

When Nate broke his arm and was "freaking out," Reagan, the cool and collected dad, gently held Nate's arm at the wrist and at the elbow and said "No, it's okay son, it's only bent... look at it." Nate, having 100% confidence in his daddy said "Really?" Reagan responded "Yes, but lets get you to the doctor and have them look at it." Of course Nate's arm was broken but as always, Reagan managed to lessen the pain greatly by applying a dose of his love, passion, and humor.

Reagan was a husband, brother, son, and a father. He was

also a police officer, a sergeant with the Las Vegas Metropolitan Police Department. Reagan worked with many officers during his tenure with the police department and, as a sergeant, he supervised many officers as well. He was a natural leader. Reagan was a flexible leader who always managed to draw the best out of everyone he worked for and everyone who worked for him. Reagan very rarely said "no" when it came to helping a fellow officer, or anyone for that matter. Reagan was a motivator and was every bit as good at multi-tasking. That is why he earned positions in some of the more prestigious positions within the agency. Reagan's last assignment with the L.V.M.P.D. was S.I.S. where he supervised a squad of police officers (detectives) who investigated business crime within Las Vegas and Clark County, Nevada. Reagan had qualities that made him a natural leader and it was those very qualities that earned him the coveted Las Vegas Metro Police Department "Life Saving Award."

Camping and fishing were two of Reagan's favorite hobbies, second only to spending time with the family. This meant fishing and camping with the family were definitely rated above simply fishing and camping. Reagan's family included God. He loved and respected his wife, Dawn, even more after 27 ½ years of marriage than he did as a young puppy in love. There was not a day that went by that Reagan did not speak of Dawn and express to others how a husband should love his wife. Reagan not only said it, he lived it. He regularly bragged about what a great wife and mother Dawn was.

Reagan held strong and close traditional values and his faith was a significant part of his life. He was a member of the Church of Christ for 28 years. During that time, Reagan enjoyed teaching Men's Bible Class as well as serving as the Youth Group Leader.

In 1986 Reagan even took a leap of faith and temporarily left the police department to serve as a full time pastor. However, he changed his mind and he returned to the police department, working as a uniformed officer. When asked why he returned to law enforcement, Reagan said "As a pastor, I found myself always asking for money. I knew that if I were to return to Metro, I could be the one financially able to help the church." Retaining his compassion for all people, Reagan and Dawn actually planned to self fund their shared missionary goals after his retirement.

Reagan loved vacationing and some of his favorite vacation spots were Big Bear Lake, Newport Beach, California and Duck Creek, Utah but if his family was with him, the location became secondary.

It goes without saying that a man who loved God and family as Reagan did, would obviously love animals... and Reagan did. The Alexander family had two cats, Pepper and Freckles but his best friend of five years was his Dachshund, Homer.

Reagan lived a full life and impacted the lives of more individuals than can ever be counted. He was honest, loving, caring and positive. He was a strong leader and an understanding and loving husband, father, brother and son. Reagan made people laugh. He made them laugh hard—gut wrenching laughs. He changed the world. He made it a better place.

On April 12, 2010, Reagan R. Alexander, an American Hero, died at his own hand in his home in Pahrump, Nevada. He will be missed but never forgotten for the world is a better place because of his contributions of which there were many.

Letter to Reagan, from Dawn Alexander (wife)

Dear Reagan,

I still cannot believe this is real. That you really took your own life. It was a shock to everyone. I do know how much pain you were in for so long, but you always persevered through it. You constantly put me and the kids first and battled through your back pain. I am so sorry that I did not know the extent of how things changed and how you were feeling so depressed and not able to handle it anymore. If only you had told me, I would have done anything to help you.

I miss you so much! You gave me 28 of the most wonderful years and I will always cherish and hold dear, the memories of a life filled with so much love. Your legacy of loving God and caring for others has touched so many and will be carried on by all who had the privilege of knowing you.

My life will never be the same without you. Now, it is my turn to persevere through the pain and I will do it with the strength God provides while holding onto the hope that I will see you again!

I love you forever,
Dawn

Letter to Reagan from his children

To our Daddy,

We know that you did not want to leave us. You made our lives wonderful and we would not be who we are without you. For so long you were in pain and we were always fine. You always took care of us, making sure that we were happy and that we had everything we needed and more. We know that, besides Christ, we were your number one priority. Now we are hurting, but for the first time in so long you are not. Finally, you are being taken care of and are able to do all the things you couldn't while on this earth.

You made us laugh; you made the best omelets, breakfast scrambles, nachos, popcorn and smoothies. Whenever there was a problem, you always made it okay. You taught us to live with integrity, and to walk with Christ. You were our baseball coach, teacher, preacher, entertainer, counselor and hero. We will miss having our Daddy here with us, but we are still a family and we cannot wait to be with you again.

We love you forever. All three!

Brandi, Nate and Caleb

Letter to Reagan from Stacy Rodd (Friend)

Reagan,

My friend, comrade and brother in Christ, do you know how much you are missed? I know that you are with angels and loved ones, and that you are with the Lord, basking in the love and peace that we spoke of when you were with us in this life. I also know that as you watch over Dawn and the kids and all of your friends and co-workers, you know the pain, anguish, torment, and confusion that losing you has brought. It is an indescribable void, this life without you. You always brought life into any room you entered with that infectious laugh, your irrepressible wit and your ability to entertain. In those funny stories you blended tales of life, work and family experiences that always drew us in and kept us laughing. I think that we all recognized your kind, gentle and humble vulnerabilities in your unique and comforting stories that became your workplace legacy. Not that there wasn't fire in your belly on occasions, we saw that too, but you always found a way to work things out amidst the crisis and get everything back on track. I think that perhaps most noteworthy was how your love and passion for God made you a living, serving saint among us. In that spirit, you always led by example, never compromising your priorities of God, family and friends in your life. That approach highlighted how an honorable, spiritually grounded and wise man proceeds through the adversity of daily existence.

You were also a tough and strong warrior who waged a valiant , lengthy and relentless battle against physical pain. We helplessly watched that battle replay itself over and over for years with little or no relief. We also saw your incomparable spirit and a tenacious will that kept you in the fight, an attribute that earned you your nickname of "The Great Silverback". Well, brother Reagan, we miss our great silverback.. We don't have our kind and caring friend who always made time for the needs of others. We don't have your strength of character to inspire us anymore. I miss our discussions of faith in service of God. I miss you.

I have to tell you though, strange little things keep your presence in our lives every day, and when I encounter these things it is bittersweet. I will laugh or smile while tears fill my eyes, and then I am overtaken by loss and despair. It is then, right then, that I will see your face, bright pink from chuckling uncontrollably, and with that vision I find peace. I realize that it is Reagan finding his way back to comfort us, and then I'm okay again. Thank you brother for coming to comfort us when we need it most.

I thank God for the brief but treasured gift of your friendship, comradery, guidance and spiritual presence in my life. We love you and miss you immensely. I smile in anticipation of laughing and sharing fellowship with you again as we have done so many times in the past. What a day that will be.

Thank you heavenly father for blessing us with our beloved brother Reagan Alexander.

Stacy Rodd

**The following letter, written by Reagan,
was recovered from the family computer
eight months after his death.**

I don't know who I am anymore. It seems I have lost something of myself. I still look out from my eyes and see a beautiful wife and awesome children. These bring me back to a purpose and a recollection of who I should be. To the great life and blessings that have been growing right in front of me for many years. But I am held back from fully embracing these blessings and I am tired of this hold on me. My joy of such a great sowing of a simple but glorious life the reaping of which is now being made bitter and confused because of my present state.

My heart wants to live a different life and to love more and do more but my body and mind are in such pain I cannot maintain order within me. I call to the One who can restore me: My heart and mind and body. I am so very tired all I have left is my voice it seems to call you and hope you will make everything alright.

Oh my God please see this wonderful sweet family—whose life is set by your existence, whose lives are yours from the time the children were conceived, whose marriage was set in your hands—and take notice of me. I want to be an example and Godly man to each... and to do that I need you to lead me to an escape from this torture! It has been long enough my God. It has been too much in my life and taken too much of our family's life.

You are my God and I am yours to do with as you please. But I know you have good for me and not bad. You have promises and not lies. I ask for your mighty hand to sweep this enemy from my castle!

I shall seek your comfort and shelter until this passes. For myself but also for my family. Please God do it soon.

Reagan

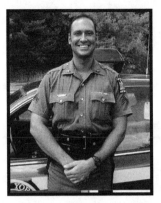

JOSEPH J. BANISH
August 4, 1972—April 1, 2008
Biography by Charlotte Banish (Mother)

Joseph James Banish was born on Friday, August 4, 1972. He was our second child but our first son. Was bald at birth, we called him bowling ball head for a year and a half, and he hated that I told people that. Anyone who knew Joe, knew how important his appearance and his hair was to him. He was yet to become the big brother of three other siblings, two who later, followed in his footsteps and became police officers. Mary, his younger sister who is now an educator, Jimmy, who is with the Washington County Sheriff's Department, and Mike, a Virginia State Trooper. Joe's oldest sister, Jennifer, is an educator as well. She teaches 4th grade at the same school they graduated from and the same school their mom still works at (FCS).

The Banish family lived in Buffalo, New York at the time of his birth, and when Joe was entering the 6th grade, moved 65 miles south to the town of Allen, New York. Joe was an athlete from an early age and began playing ice hockey as a small boy in Buffalo. Joe graduated from Fillmore Central School in 1990. He followed his older sister Jennifer, to Saint Bonaventure University where he graduated a Pre-Law/Philosophy Major.

When Joe was a little boy, a large branch broke off the tree in front of the house and he said "Don't worry, dad can tape it." He always thought tape could fix the world. He also had a little green hang truck, as he called it. (It was a tow truck but it had two hooks on the back so Joe called it his "Hang Truck.")

Even as a small boy, Joe loved the game of golf and one time while playing at the 6S Golf Course, he took a few too many swings on the first hole and the owner shouted "One practice swing." Joe got older and loved his Ford Mustang and later enjoyed his Black F150 every bit as much. Joe was a scout in his younger years and his scoutmaster was a retired serviceman who taught the boys how to repel down hills, survive the outdoors, and sleep out on Cuba Lake. He came home frozen as a popsicle but he received his Ice Mole Badge for it.

When Joe cultivated a friendship with someone it lasted for life. Kenny graduated from the academy with Joe and was like a brother to him. In fact, Joe always referred to him as his brother. Ronnie and Carl were two of those life long friends and their relationships began in high school. Ronnie was at Joe's house constantly. In fact, he was there so often that Joe's mom, Char, used to call Ronnie her fourth son. On one occasion later in their lives, Joe and Ronnie were caught in a snow storm coming home from Olean. Their car was stuck and when they got out of it in an attempt to "unstick it," there was a deer standing behind the car. The car then began to slide down the hill. Both Joe and Ronnie had to shout at the deer to get out of the way because it was in the path of the car sliding down the hill. It was one of his funniest stories, and everyone listening laughed whenever Joe told the story.

Another of Joe's very good friends was Dave, aka Brownie, and Joe loved hunting with him. Joe used to tell stories about Brownie that made him sound as if he were Rambo and how Brownie could hunt as Rambo hunted. Whenever they went hunting, Brownie never came home empty handed.

During college at St. Bonaventure, Joe worked as a counselor at the Jim Kelley Football Camp, which was held at the Bonaventure Campus for a few years. His brother Jimmy, who was four years younger, asked Joe if he could work with him, so Joe gave his brother's name to the person in charge. Jimmy received his rejection letter in the mail stating that he was only 17 and didn't have enough driving experience to drive the football celebrities around. Jimmy called Joe and Joe then wrote a letter to the person in charge, singing Jim's praises and a few weeks later, Jimmy had the job. Jimmy then received a letter from the person in charge stating he had received a letter from Joe telling him what a fantastic person Jimmy was. The letter stated that Jimmy was not only trustworthy, but highly experienced. Jimmy ended up making more money than Joe did that year because he earned such great tips from the celebrities. Joe constantly teased him about that! Jimmy never lived it down.

Upon graduation from college, Joe immediately knew he wanted to be part of the State Police Family. He took the test and was admitted to the very next class. He attended the police academy from November 28, 1993, his dad's birthday, and graduated on May 26, 1994, the day before his mom's birthday.

This was a very special event and a day of great pride for the entire family. One evening when he was able to phone home from the academy, Joe's mother, Charlotte (Char) Banish, told him how very proud the entire family was of him. She told Joe they were proud of his being accepted to the academy, how hard he was working and studying and how excited they were about and couldn't wait for his graduation. Char didn't realize that Joe had already spoken with his sister Jen and told her that he had packed his bag, and was calling to announce that he was coming home... He didn't think this job was for him after all. Things changed however, after mom talked to Joe, telling him how proud everyone was. They changed because Joe went back to his room, unpacked his bag, and decided to "tough it out" so he wouldn't disappoint his family.

Joe Banish was stationed at various stations throughout his career and his family often teased him about going right through the alphabet of stations. Joe became an investigator and then decided he could be a much better trooper as a sergeant so, he took the exam, passed it, and became one of the youngest sergeants with the State Police at that time. The young Sergeant Banish so enjoyed being a commanding officer that he took the lieutenant's exam, scoring 7th on the raw score.

Studying for the lieutenant's exam took six months and as part of studying for that test, Joe made audio tapes to listen to in the car as he drove back and forth to work. Joe also made index cards for studying, so many cards in fact that his mother would often tease him stating that had she known how many index cards he would have been using in his life time, she would have bought stock in them.

Joe earned the Trooper Patrol Award, was an FTO (Field Training Officer), and a pistol expert. He was a real marksman and loved target shooting. He treasured all of his guns.

When he took the promotional exam for Lieutenant, Joe's family teased him relentlessly about the movie *Dances With Wolves* because there was one scene in the movie when the Indian Chief had a conversation with Kevin Costner (who played a lieutenant in the movie) and called him "lieutenttant." Joe's family could not wait for him to promote so they could call him lieutenttant.

Joe loved being with his family. He would often return home and target shoot with his father and brothers, ride 4 wheelers on their 60 acres of land, vacation with family, and enjoy to no end, being with his two brothers, two sisters and nine nieces and nephews. Hawaii and Myrtle Beach were Joe's two favorite vacation spots but he was every bit as happy camping with family up in the Adirondack Mountains.

Joe and the rest of the family vacationed together in Hawaii for his parents' 30th wedding anniversary. The family still, and will forever, cherish the memories of scuba diving, drinking mai tais, and cooking their own steaks at the Outrigger with Joe and Dawn. Joe loved every family vacation and he loved the many train excursions he went on with the family. He truly enjoyed riding over the Letchworth State Park Bridge on one of the trips as that bridge held special childhood memories for him and the rest of the family (memories of family picnics when the entire family would walk out onto the high bridge).

Joe's favorite holidays were Christmas and the 4th of July. Christmas was special because as much as he loved giving gifts, he loved getting them. He loved Christmas goodies, being together with everybody, and going to church on Christmas Eve with family. When Joe first became an altar boy in the 4th grade, he served midnight mass and that was really special to him. Joe had to hang his ornament highest on the tree every Christmas; Family always teased him about that. In fact, he always had to be first to do everything in the family. As his mother says, "Now he's the first to be in heaven, paving the way for all of us I'm sure, standing at the pearly gates, waiting to welcome us in."

Joe called New Year's Eve at the Banish Family House "Rockin' Eve." The family had so much fun together and they always had pizza and wings to bring in the New Year.

Joe was so fussy that he wouldn't eat the skin on the wings or the veins in the wings and if you have ever eaten chicken wings, you know that doesn't leave much to eat.

The Banish family always vacationed for a week during the 4th of July. This was an entire week that the family spent together and did nothing but family stuff. The men would target shoot, golf, swim, drink, grill and eat. The girls would do everything else. For a short time Joe owned a boat and kept it at Bristol Mountain in Canandaigua. What fun the family had speeding up and down the lake in that boat. Joe was called the "Grillmeister" at all of the cookouts and Joe's sister-in-law, Tasha, even took a photo of him at the grill with smoke wafting through the air. She framed it, put stickers around the frame (because of his "Do I look like a clown" saying) and gave it to him for Christmas. Joe loved gifts like that and when he opened the gift, responded with another one of his trademark statements... "Nicely done."

Joe loved peanut brittle, particularly his mother's brittle that she made during the holidays. Joe would eat all of his and come back for more. He also loved cookies with Hershey's kisses on top (he could go through an entire batch in one sitting). Joe, as an adult, learned that his mom could still bake pastry hearts just like the ones he ate as a kid. The last time Joe was at his mother's house, Holy Saturday, he ate about a dozen of the pastry hearts and asked if she could bake more next time he came over.

Joe used to make his girlfriend, Dawn, repeat sayings about his uncle Bob, over and over until none of us could stand it! They were hysterical. There was always "Fishy Birdie" and the relentless fan he had to have on at night. He loved horseshoes, going to the 'H,' biking on the canal, cakes on the griddle, his wet suit (and trying to get into it after gaining a few pounds), Napoleon, bowling at the Pines, playing Medal of Honor all night long on the computer with Mike, his battery operated toothbrush (and lecturing his nieces and nephews on dental health), whistling "Feliz Navidad," named two flies at Jen's house, Ted and Frank, the "No Fly Zone" for the crows, Operation Deer Slayer, calling Chad, Dennis, shooting clays at Jen and Chris' house.

Joe Banish was a beautiful man. He was just as beautiful on the inside as he was on the outside. He had a heart of gold. In fact, Joe was generous to a fault. He would give people the shirt off his back and many times he did. Joe loved helping people. He gave many of his belongings away after he bought them or wouldn't buy himself anything unless he first purchased one for his brothers and one for his father. He thought, or at least wanted, everyone to live to be 100.

Joe idolized his father and always wanted to be just like him. He was so proud of his dad being a Town Justice and his mom being a court clerk. When his dad ran for office one term, Joe passed out his dad's campaigning pens to his trooper buddies in Binghamton and Bath who kept asking for more.

Joe loved Sugarland and all country music. Joe's mom even got him to a couple of Kenney Chesney concerts. Some of his favorite drinks included Heineken, Pepsi, and White Grape Juice. He loved his cats, Kimber and Miles. He loved Olive Garden, Outback Steakhouse, and BOCES Pizza on Clinton Street. (He even talked his friends from the casino into getting pizza from there when he was an investigator in Niagara Falls.) He also loved Red Lobster, The Buffalo Sabers, and the Mets. He loved every Al Pacino film (*Heat* was his favorite).

Joe's mother and father dedicated him to the Blessed Mother at his baptism and Joe maintained his devotion to her throughout his life. Joe had a true devotion to the rosary and said it daily.

These were only two more reasons out of thousands that fueled Joe's mother's pride. Char could not have been more proud of Joe, and his actions and beliefs throughout his life are some of the moments she quotes when saying she knows he was met by the blessed mother when he arrived at the gates to heaven.

Joe was very proud of being a state trooper and he was involved in so many aspects of the agency. He even played ice hockey as an adult just as he did as a child, only now , he played for the State Police Troop C Flames. He was also proud of his faith. There is nothing quite like seeing a strapping 238 pound man in a state police lieutenant's uniform who was never ashamed of his faith nor was he ashamed to show it.

Joe Banish was a very handsome man and many of his friends had nicknames for him. Some called him "Hollywood," some called him "Long Island Lolita" and some called him "Trooper Chippendale" (his mom's favorite). Joe wasn't the only one with nicknames though. Joe had nicknames for his friends and family. He called his mom "The Cooler" because she could always calm everything down. His dad was "Big Duke Six" because they enjoyed watching *Apocalypse Now* together. There was also "Scoob," Dutchie, Pig Pen, Little Ladies, Kringle, Mamsie, Jiambi, Neichie, Jibs, Kenny Shamrock, Little Frank, Nip Nooger, The Goofball Brothers, Little Chum, and Little Buddy just to name a few.

Joe loved clowning around and whenever he would do something silly, he would ask, "Do I look like a clown to you?" which made it even funnier. As a gag gift for Christmas, Joe's mom bought him a clown nose which he thought hilarious. One of the family's most treasured photos of Joe is one of him wearing the clown nose.

Joe was the perfect son and on one Mother's Day, he sent his mother a Mother's Day Email rather than a card. In the email, he told his mother that he wanted to show his love and feelings for his mom in his words, not the words of someone else. The email made Char cry for half a day. Joe always sent cards and emails and in every one he said that his mother was the one who held his family together.

At the time of Joe's death, he was a Lieutenant at the academy in Albany, New York, the place he wanted to be. Joe Banish loved being a trooper. It was his entire life. Joe put off having a family to study and move up the ladder first so he wouldn't take time away from his family later. Joe's plan was to then have a wife and children and dedicate his life to them. Unfortunately, Joe never married and he never had any children. His family has only memories and photos. No grand children, nieces, or nephews.

Lieutenant James Joseph Banish a beautiful and wonderful human being, an American Hero, died at his own hand in New York on Tuesday April 1, 2008.

Upon Joe's death, the family found a box that had the words "Important Papers" written on it. Inside that box, among many items, was his clown nose his mother had given to him as a gag gift. On October 24, 2008, six months after Joe's death, his brother Mike and Mike's wife, Tasha, had a baby boy. They named him Joseph. When Joe was a little boy, he couldn't pronounce his name and said "Jofus." Now, Alex, Mike and Tasha's other son, call his little brother "Jofus."

When the first anniversary of Joe's death neared, his mother asked family members to write 35 memories of Joe (he was 35 years old at death). The entire family attended Mass that April 1st and then went to the cemetery in the pouring rain to remember and share memories. This was a beautiful way for family to memorialize Joe. Family members cried as they remembered Joe and the nieces and nephews remembered: dancing on Uncle Joe's feet at Uncle Mike's wedding, kiss time for the little ladies, how he called everyone "Little Buddy," how he loved everyone, clown school, he was so fun to be with, how he was so awesome at being awesome, how their ticket into his house was telling him that he was their favorite uncle.

Joe's family members miss him more than words can say. Survive Joe!

Letter to Joe from Charlotte Banish (Mother)

My dear son Joe,

I can honestly say that I never thought I would be writing a letter to you telling you how very much you are missed. Naturally, it is not normal for a child to die before their parents, and I never thought I would be standing in these shoes. I can't tell you how much I miss you. How I miss your jokes, your big larger than life smile, your side kisses, your visits, your just calling to say "Hi mom, just calling to see how you are." I miss you in the summer, at strawberry picking time when you would come to visit, and I would have homemade strawberry shortcake. You would tell me you must have gained 10 pounds that day because the bowl never left your hand for the entire time you were home.

I miss our Fourth of July week long vacations. I miss you talking dad into going golfing, then calling him "David Hasselhoff" from *Bay Watch* because you told dad he spent more time in the sand than David did! I miss you target shooting with dad even though you guys would sometimes ruin a perfectly good tree with bullets. I miss our annual excursions on the Miss Buffalo boat trip. I loved how you called me "The Cooler" and dad "Big Duke." I loved how you had nicknames for everyone! I miss you in the Fall and our visits up to your land on a beautiful Fall Day. You would be planning your strategy for hunting, and telling everyone where they would be located on opening day, you even bought Dad a heater for the blind because you didn't want him to freeze. You were so very proud of that land and loved riding your four wheelers up there. You even talked your brothers into buying four wheelers also so you all could ride together and what fun you all had up there. I miss you on opening day at lunch time and after eating your chili, you taking a nap instead of going back out in the woods.

I miss you in the Winter because you loved Christmas. Your ornament always had to be the highest on the tree, but that was okay with everyone because they knew that was important to you! You were such a giver at Christmas, but you also loved receiving. And I miss you in the Spring when your flower garden is in full bloom. I planted a little "Joey's garden" from the bulbs and plants that people sent for your funeral. It is really beautiful and I know you would love it!

I guess I miss you all the time Joe. I miss what could have been, your wedding, your children, God knows they would have been knockouts! I miss the fun we were yet to have together. The good times and yes, even the bad. We were a family and we shared it all, and got through it all together! I know that your friends also miss you. So many of them spoke to me at the funeral parlor or sent me letters telling me just how important you were to them. How you had an impact on their lives and some even told me you impacted their children.

You gave one officer a booklet on how to pray the rosary for his son. Your friends wear the bracelets we had made in your memory. *"In memory of NYSP Lieutenant Joseph J. Banish 1899 April 1, 2008."* None of us will ever forget you Joe.

So many of your friends told me funny stories about SPSP, how they wondered who exactly was enjoying the water park more, you or the under privileged kids you took there. Stories that revealed you as the hero you are Joe, even though your name will never appear on the wall at the Academy. You were a hero to so many, most of all because we knew what was in your heart.

You had a heart of gold and a smile that lit up an entire room. You had such a presence and turned every head as you entered! I miss your big beautiful brown eyes! God blessed our lives and the world when He made you. Whatever you did, you did it the best! You had to; it was who you were. We will forever love and cherish your memory, all that you were and all that you will be forever in our hearts.

Remember when you were in kindergarten, and like so many little kids who can't fit their entire name on the front of an art project, you wrote JOSE on the front, I looked on the back for the PH but it wasn't there and we joked about us now having a new son named "Jose," which I continued to call you sometimes through the years.

After you died, the first time I saw your truck in our yard, I thought your death was a horrible dream, and for just the slightest second, I thought you were still here. I wanted to yell up to dad, "Hon, Joe is here." How I wish you could have told us what was going on at work. We would have helped you, you could still be here with us.

Where are you Joe? Why aren't you here? I ask myself that every day. You were my first little boy and there was always a special bond between us. You never did anything without checking with us first. You always valued our opinion. You never wanted to do anything wrong, or that would shame your family. You were too perfect. You always made us so very proud of your accomplishments! I thank God for every day that we had you here on earth. I treasure all the wonderful memories of my beautiful son!

I know that you are in heaven, waiting and getting things ready for our arrival. You always took care of our entire family in some way.

Not only my heart, but also the hearts of our entire family are beyond repair. We are all so broken. A spoke from our family wheel is missing and cannot be repaired. How can we go on without you Joe? Some days I don't want to, and wish I didn't have to. I wish God would call me home so that we could have dinner together tonight. I miss you so much. I guess I can't tell you that enough.

People keep telling me that things will get better. Nothing is better, or even close to it. No days are good, some are bearable, all are bad without you. I go through the motions of life, of holidays, for everyone else, but truly my life is never going to be the same.

I was very glad I chose to speak at your funeral. I hope you were proud of the things that I said and that I was able to tell everyone what a wonderful son you are. So many people asked me how I could speak at my son's funeral, my answer was "How could I not." How could I not take the last opportunity to tell the entire church, full of friends, family and State Police Officers, how much we miss you, and how much we love you and always will.

Remember the day Mike graduated from the Virginia State Police Academy? It was one of the proudest days of my life when you and Jimmy were able to hand Mike his diploma. My three beautiful sons on the stage as police officers. I remember when they introduced Jimmy as a Washington County Deputy Sheriff, and then you as a sergeant in the NY State Police, everyone said "Wow!" Boy, did that do a mother's heart good. I was so proud!

Your nieces and nephews talk about you constantly. There is not a visit, or a holiday that we don't talk about Uncle Joe. The boys miss hunting with you. They all miss your jokes, your teasing, your nick names, your reminding them to brush and floss their teeth every time they saw you. They miss everything about you. You were so loved Joe, how did you not know that we could get through anything together, considering all our family has already been through? We are such a close family. You used to tease everyone and tell them nothing was a secret once one of us knew something, telling us "It would be around the horn" in seconds. Why didn't you tell us how hurt and worried you were?

I will end this letter to you Joe, telling you yet once more, that you were and still are so loved by your family. I pray that the time until we meet again is short. I pray that God has mercy on your soul and the souls of our family and friends, so that we may all meet together in heaven and have yet one more of our big beautiful family reunions where we will be separated no more and I can hear you clap your hands the way only you could, and say "I love it."

I remember the last time I talked to you on the phone. After you talked to dad, you wanted to speak to me. I asked you if you were watching *Dancing With The Stars* because both you and I loved that show. You told me "No" because you were going to bed because you were very tired but you just wanted to say goodnight and tell me that you loved me. Those were the last words I ever heard you speak. You always ended every conversation to all of us with "I love you." You were such a loving son.

My precious son, how I wished you would have reached out to me that morning. I would have told you to come home, all would have been well, and we are here, always.

I love you Joe, and will for all eternity. Rest in peace "Little Buddy" my beautiful son. You never said "I'm leaving;" you never said "Goodbye." Yet you were gone before I knew it and only God knows why.

A million times I needed you; a million times I've cried if love alone could have saved you, you never would have died. In life, I loved you dearly, in death, I love you still. In my heart you hold a place that no one else can fill. I love you so my precious son and I always will. It broke my heart to lose you but you didn't go alone, for part of me went with you the day God called you home. The years stretch on before me so bleak and dark and long. I pray you walk beside me son and help to keep me strong. And when my life is over, come to me on that day and smile at me and hold me tight and carry me away. The wind that whispers through the trees, the brightest stars at night, a rainbow on a dismal day, a ray of golden light. All these are signs you send to me, a message from above that even death can't break the bonds of a Son and a Mother's love.

Mom XXXOOO

Letter to Joe from his Dad

Joe,

We had good times hunting on your land. Do you remember the time we went down the icy road and had the two ATVs and the truck jackknifed across the road? After getting the truck and trailer headed down the hill, we went on to hunt. That was the last time we hunted together.

We enjoyed going to breakfast together after morning mass or just meeting you at breakfast from time to time. We did so many wonderful things together and I miss you so much Joe. I really loved golfing with you, even though you used to make fun of my being in the sand, and having more time in there than David Hasselhoff!

Your help was much appreciated around the house by plowing snow, building the garage, bringing in wood or pellets (4-40lb bags at a time) or just helping fix the cars. I remember a day of wood cutting to clear trails for the ATVs. The trails are still there, and we treasure them.

There are many more things that I think of from time to time but I have an extremely hard time writing about them now because the loss of my son is hard to bare. We will be together again Joe, until that time, remember that Big Duke loves you with all of his heart. Rest in peace little buddy!

Love, Dad

Letter to Joe from Jen (Sister)

Dear Joe,

It is so difficult for me to write you this letter, because by writing it, I feel that you will respond back to me.

Joe, You have touched my life and the lives of everyone in my family—Chris and, of course, the kids in so many ways. There is not a single day that goes by that there's not a special mention made of "Uncle Joe" in my home. It pains me to see Zach, Elliott, Lizzie, and Tara growing up into adults without the person who made a positive, lasting impression in each and every one of their lives in a very wonderful way. Please know Joe, that Elliott and Zach have treasured every waking moment that they have spent with you and have become avid hunters because of you. Know too, that Lizzie and Tara loved when you teased them and played around with them.

I have a picture of you and me together on my wedding day, its sitting next to my bed. I look at this picture every night before I go to bed. Joe, that was one of the happiest days of my life. But when I look at the picture and the smiles on our faces, dancing together, I smile to myself and then just as fast I find myself getting teary-eyed and I can't help but think of how sad, and incomplete our family is now, without your presence. You were a very large part of our family get-togethers. I especially miss hearing your laugh at the kitchen table, as you, Jimmy and Mike reminisced about things you did as kids. I miss your smile as you walked through the door upon entering my home. I miss your cute little nicknames for everyone, your dental floss, and your white T-shirts. Our many memories of you keep you here with us, close by.

Our memories are all we have... Thank God, there are many, many, happy memories, all including you. I am proud to be your sister and I am proud of all your many accomplishments in your life. You are truly an honorable person, brother, and police officer.

Joe, I know you are watching over us. You are a special angel. I know you are in heaven, pain free and at peace. One of the only thoughts that keep me going is knowing that I will see you again, someday. Until then...

All my love.

Jen

Letter to Joe from Mary (Sister)

Joe,

Kid, I just want to start by telling you how much I miss you, and how I wish you were still here! I don't think you could have ever realized how much losing you impacted our family... especially mom. I'm getting married this year, and it really saddens me to know you won't be there. I remember Jen and Mike's weddings. How much fun we all had dancing and singing. The thing I remember most is when you danced the hand jive. It was so hilarious to watch you run around the floor doing the Lasso move. It breaks my heart to know that when I have more children, they will never have the honor of meeting their Uncle Joe or knowing first hand what a genuine man you were. All of your nieces and nephews will do an outstanding job telling stories about you because anyone you came in contact with was truly blessed by knowing you.

I just want to go through some memories that often go through my mind when I think about you. The first one is when we lived in Scoville and we weren't allowed to cross the street, but we did anyway because you wanted to go see Tracy Catanzaro. While we were there two boys started a fight with you, and you asked me for help, so I beat one of the boys up, and we walked home laughing and trying to make up a story to tell mom so we wouldn't get in trouble. Another one is when we used to bowl together at the Rose Bowl Lanes, and how we dreaded getting up on Saturday mornings, but we always had so much fun!

I remember when we were in high school and mom allotted us each a certain amount of time for the bathroom in the morning, and how you and your hair took up so much time that you would cut into all our time, and we would argue, but you still stayed in front of the mirror, and then we would have to walk out to the front for the bus and you would walk into the wind so you wouldn't mess up your hair. I remember when the mailman used to give us Tic Tacs, and when he didn't have any, we would wait until he went by and then put the flag up so he would have to stop on the way down the hill as we hid in the tree by the road laughing!

I remember all the good times we had while we were in college. We would eat breakfast, lunch and dinner together every day, and you would eat the Captain Crunch with the Crunch Berries in it for most of your meals, and would pick out all the cereal and throw it on the tray and eat just the Crunch Berries. I remember when you, me, Dawn, and Ronnie went on spring break and we got so sun burned on our faces and when we got back we couldn't find anyone, and we thought it was the rapture so we decided to go to Jen's because we knew she would still be here, and we scared her half to death because of the blisters from the sunburn.

You know, I looked forward to your State Police Stories because you had a way of making things so funny! Like the time you and Jimmy changed a family's transmission in the dead of winter because they were stuck on the side of the road.

There are so many things that I remember like going to our proms together, we would make ice cream sundaes after church on Saturday nights and yours would always be the biggest. How when we would decorate the Christmas tree, you would always put your Blue Joey ornament on the top. How you would wear those thick black belts when you were a little boy and how you truly believed tape fixed everything; luckily, dad had a big supply of it.

I remember how when we would go out to the country for the weekend, we would beg dad to stop at the Jenny Lee Dairy, and just because you asked last and he stopped, you would say "Thanks to me, we're eating ice cream." I remember when we were watching Rambo and you sat on the stove and burned your butt. And whenever you got your hair cut, you would cry. When mom and dad would drag us apple picking and we would hate going but when we got there we had so much fun climbing trees. I remember when mom used to dress you, me, and Jen alike when we were little... those Mickey Mouse outfits and the "Squeeze Me" shirts.

I remember working at Little Caesar's and we would throw ham at each other and try to make it stick on each other's face, and you would always get a kick out of when Mr. Johnson would pull up and hold 2 fingers up and I would ignore him and make him walk in to order. I remember when you worked at J.C. Penney and had to walk to work from Bonaventure. I remember the time we went Trick-or-Treating down that long driveway and mom waited at the end and after we got our candy, we scared Mike and ran as fast as we could to the van and Mike was too little to keep up and when he was running, he dragged his bag and all his candy came out on the driveway, but we were all too scared to get out and get it. I remember the spook houses we did, when we would dress up in the cassocks from church.

Jen and I still laugh about the time you took Lady out in the back yard and we listened for a shot but never heard one... then we saw you walking back with Lady trotting behind you. I remember when you and Jen put those plastic clogs on me and put baby oil on mom and dad's bedroom floor and shoved me in and I couldn't stand up. I remember when I called you for help and you ran around the building with your chest puffed out.

I remember doing Freshman Orientation at Bonaventure and how much fun we had. I really miss all those times we had and remember them so vividly. It seems like just yesterday that we were going out in college. I miss the fact that we would talk every year on our birthdays, even when you wouldn't answer for other people.

I remember you making up a crazy story telling dad that I worked for Aladdin's Limousine because they couldn't figure out where the shirt came from. I remember going to the John Denver Concert and how we could see his back the entire time. I remember working at the chicken farm together, riding to school with you when you drove your senior year, going to school at St. Bernard's, those crazy times with Alicia Schwabb, Nicole Blachura, and Lisa and Jeff Wawrzyniak. Like when we would ring the Young's doorbell and run away, and making mud pies for the dumb boys in the back. I remember when you and Jimmy lived in the "Sugar Shack/Sugar Shanty."

I remember when we were little and we would play hide and seek in the other room with the huge toy box and you would try to make us laugh by saying "Poopy Lock" and when we would laugh, you could find us. There are so many memories to reflect on and I feel so robbed that we won't be able to make any more. Kid, we all love you so much, I just wish I would have known you felt so overwhelmed. I feel like I could have helped you if only I knew. You know, your picture is the screen saver to my Blackberry and I still talk to you all the time. I just wish you were here to hear me.

Rest in peace little buddy, I love you!!!

Min

Letter to Joe from Jimmy (Brother)

Joey,

Hey Baugh!!! I first wanted to say I miss you. It's awfully lonely down here without the happiness you used to bring to everyone. Since you left, nothing is the same. I still try to call you every morning, afternoon, and night, only to realize that after I dial your number, you aren't going to answer. It breaks my heart knowing that I never get to see your smile, or hear your wonderful laugh again. Some days I used to wonder how many times you would call me throughout the day and it would usually be 5 or 6. Then again, I would reciprocate and do the same to you. What I wouldn't do for just one more of those calls when we talk about nothing, but it meant everything.

Domanic asks often about Uncle Joe and asks what exactly happened to you. Everyone knows he is "The Golden Child" in your eyes, and I don't know what to tell him. He is very sad, especially when we talk about you and recall all of the wonderful memories. You would be so proud of him, he hit a home run in All Stars this year. I wish you could have seen him. He made the sign of the cross and said it was for his Uncle Joe and looked into the sky and pointed to you. He told me before every game this year that he was going to do good for his Uncle Joe and he explained to me how you helped him pitch and hit from heaven. He misses you more than you will ever know. He is getting so tall and he even looks like you, even more now.

We often get a chuckle talking about last year when you were in my house for Dom's birthday and I told him that he was too young for a bb-gun, and as usual, he talked to you and you took him to WalMart and bought him the gun. Dom even eats like you, just as fussy and picks apart his food. I don't even say anything to him, I just sit back and marvel in the likeliness. Jarrett or "Pop tart" as you used to call him, reminds me every time he sees your picture in my bedroom, that you used to call him "Pop tart" and lets out a little chuckle. He too has gotten very big and even as young as he was when you left us, he still asks where you are to which we explain that you live with Jesus now. It usually sparks a sigh and the perpetual question, "Why don't you ask Jesus if we can have him back?" I am just thankful that he has so many memories and had gotten the chance to know you even as brief as it was. All fathers could only hope that their children will turn out even half as well as you did. Please look over them and help to guide them in your likeliness. Mom and dad are lost without you, to say the least. The once perfect family now has a hole in it bigger than the one that sank the Titanic. If not for their faith, they would have jumped in with you. They have been so strong and helped to keep the family together since we lost you. You never realized how important you were to our family. You were the stable ground in all of our lives, we always turned to you when shit went bad. You always had the answers that could fix the problem, kid. If only you could have seen the ramifications to your family, I'm sure you would still be here.

Dad, Mike, Zach and I went up to your property and I got my first deer this year. I know you would have loved it and it showed the validity of buying that land for hunting and 4 wheeling. It was the first time I went hunting since you left us. Dom just got his hunting license and can't wait to go hunting on Uncle Joe's land. We are going to spend some time this summer at your beloved property. I know how much you loved it so we are going to take good care of it.

Brandy and I finally got married after all. We had a beautiful wedding on the beach in Key West most of our families came to celebrate. We brought your picture along so you could be there too. You were the best man and I felt you there alongside me throughout the entire day. I remember how we used to talk about getting married when we were kids laying in bed and trying to decide who was going to be who's best man. You got to be Mike's and I got to be yours, and you were mine. I used to love the many world changing conversations we used to enjoy in bed as children while mom and dad thought we were sleeping. Remember the Nerf Basketball in the bedroom, the countless Wiffle Ball games, Pumpkin Football, Operation Deer Slayer, burning the ants, Matchbox Car cities, and G.I.Joe? There are so many great memories with you. I wish we had more time here to make more of those memories, but obviously, God had a greater need for you. I'm sorry for anything I ever did that made you mad at me. I want to thank you for being the big brother that I needed to get through life. Lets face it, we all know I wouldn't be here today if it weren't for you. Thanks for teaching me how to be a man and how to help others in need, even when I didn't want to. Thanks for always being there when I needed you. Thanks for being the most awesome big brother ever.

I remember the cold nights living in Westport and sleeping in the same bed because we didn't have enough money for fuel, and praying the Rosary together as we shivered, yet you still thanked God for everything we had.

The year I was in college and you paid for my books because

I wasn't working and I would call mom and ask her how to make chili so we could stretch our dollar. Those times forged a bond between us that would never be broken. You always included me in everything you did and I thank you for that. Thanks again for paying my way to Spring Break that year just so I could be with you. Remember the Magnum P.I. shorts we made and singing California Love as loud as we could, with the windows down in Daytona Beach? What about the Jim Kelly Football Camp? I never would have gotten that job if it weren't for you... Even though I made more money than you did. I did make it up to you though by taking you anywhere you wanted to go in the 15 passenger van they gave me. Of course, that included, picking you and Ronnie up last from the bars so you could drink longer than everyone else. And, don't forget the 4:00 AM smoke shows in the parking lot of RIT, just for the fun of it. I loved driving by you in the Cushman and waving as you ran with the kids. Thanks for helping me become a police officer. I wouldn't be on the job without you, in fact, the only reason I became a police officer was to be like you. Thanks for all the times we shared together big brother, good and bad. I'm glad I had the chance to write to you one last time, Joey, I have cried every day since you left. My heart actually aches because I miss you so much. One of the hardest times is when I am at Mass and it's time for Communion. I remember when I was too young to receive and told you how I wanted to go up and get it and how badly I wanted to try it. Of course, I wasn't allowed and stayed behind in the seat and waited for everyone to return from the Altar. To my surprise, when you came back, you motioned for me to be quiet and opened your mouth and broke a piece of the eucharist off for me. You just winked and smiled at me as I ate the bread. Even then you were taking care of me. That memory has stayed with me all of these years and still today, I break down and cry after receiving Communion. I will carry on here on earth for the time being, thankful for the time the Lord gave us with you. I will try to be a good father to my children and will speak often of you. I will prepare them and myself for the day in which we will see you again. I will honor you with my actions here on earth and remember the kindness you bestowed upon us, but until that day comes, just remember I LOVE YOU MY BROTHER. Watch over us all.

Love Always, Jimmy aka Baugh

Letter to Joe from Mike (Brother)

My brother Joe was a unique person, brother, and idol. As far back as I can remember, I have always looked up to Joe and tried to shadow his every move. Joe was kind, easy to talk to, soft hearted, and always looked out for his family members. He was well groomed and always worried about how presentable he looked. Every day I put on my duty belt , it reminds me of Joe. One night I was on a ride along with him and we went to breakfast at about 3:00 AM. We both exited the Tahoe and if you knew Joe, he lifted up his belt and pointed forward as if Mr. Cool had just arrived on scene. As you all know in the law enforcement community, your duty belt always moves around on your waist and it never settles to where you're comfortable. Every time I saw Joe after that , I always reminded him of that moment and now I find myself doing the same thing every morning.

Joe welcomed me into the law enforcement family when I graduated from my state basic school in 2004 and it was the greatest day in the world. I felt like I was untouchable because I had my big brother, a sergeant with the New York State Police, hand me my diploma on stage, in front of all of my fellow law enforcement brothers. Boy was that awesome. Joe was the primary reason why I entered the law enforcement field because he always reminded me of how great of a job it was. No two days were the same and you could drive around rather than be stuck behind a desk doing the same thing day after day.

There are numerous memories of Joe in my head and all of them are equally important. The biggest one that stands out is the time when he saved my life. It was always talked about amongst us three brothers... About buying ATVs and riding around on Joe's land. Joe, once again helped me by going and looking at an ATV that Jim found and called me immediately to tell me to purchase it. Needless to say, I purchased the ATV and a date was set for us three brothers to go and have some fun. As the day went on with excessive fun, all three of us started riding more aggressively. At that time, Joe stopped and mentioned that if we were going to ride that hard, we should go back to the truck and put our helmets on. Joe was just a safe person and was worried about one of us getting hurt. Sure enough, about 10 minutes later, I went over a 35 foot embankment and my ATV landed on top of me. The back of my head struck a tree stump and I blacked out for a moment. If it hadn't been for Joe, the big brother that I looked up to and listened to, I'm sure I would have died that day. My big brother saved my life.

Joe was an avid hunter, gun enthusiast, golfer, and hockey player. Whenever we four guys would get together, Joe and I were partners. I remember July 4th weekend, 2007, we had a horse shoe tournament at my sister Jen's house. Once again, Joe and I were paired up and he came up with a move that was only used when either of us threw a ringer. We would run towards each other and jump in the air, back to back. It was unknown why we did this but it is something I laugh about constantly when I play shoes. He was my best man in my wedding and welcomed my wife, Tasha, into the family.

When Tasha and I first started dating, Joe and his fiancé, Dawn, were warm welcoming Tasha and found out fast that we enjoyed going on his boat and relaxing on Canandaigua Lake. He trusted me so much that he made me a key for the boat but also reinforced that I was not to drive unless he was there. That was Joe, always taking care of me but also keeping in mind, his big brother responsibilities. After a nice hot day on the water, they always treated us to dinner back at the apartment. The one thing I couldn't stand was eating tomatoes and Joe always made me eat them. What he did was put diced tomatoes in a salad, told me they were good for me and that I didn't have a choice. It was our ongoing joke that whatever he said, went.

Joe was such an influence in my life and in my decisions; I made him my oldest son, Alex's godfather and left him to Joe in our will. Joe was so happy that he was a godfather of a boy that I never heard the end of it. He always spoke of what sort of toy we could all play with. You see, with Joe, the child inside him never left and when he bought a toy for Alex, he also got one for himself so we all could play. You can see how caring Joe was because he was so excited about the gift. He told me that I could guess what the toy was but Joe always had to give hints. I guessed correctly before Christmas but he wouldn't tell me it was the right guess; he didn't want to ruin the surprise for both Alex and I. It was a police car decorated with NYSP magnets.

In honor of Joe, and to show how much I respected him, I named my second son, Joseph, after his uncle Joe that same year. We now have another Joseph in the family and I pray to the Lord our Father that he is like his uncle, caring, loving, respectful, intelligent, and more importantly, that he puts his family first like Joe did.

My brother Joe had an influence on so many people in this world and I thank God every day that he was my brother. I wish Joe was back here calling me on my cell phone just to say "Hi" or meeting him at mom and dad's house just to hang out. He has been one of my biggest inspirations in my life and I would listen to whatever he had to say. That amazing young man always pointed me in the right direction, gave me great advice, and always kept me out of harm's way. You couldn't ask for a better big brother than Lt. Joseph J. Banish-1899 forever.

Exerpts from letters written to Joe by his nieces and nephew

A person I admire, by Zach Austin:

The person I admire most is my Uncle Joe Banish. At every family gathering he would play with his nieces and nephews instead of talking with the adults. Uncle Joe's favorite saying was "That's a fact" and he loved saying that after you said something he had never heard before. When he would buy presents for my sisters, Lizzie and Tara, he would say "Kiss time for the little ladies." Uncle Joe's best saying was "Do I look like a clown to you?" and he would say it when someone did or said something stupid. Uncle Joe could let you know you were being silly without making you feel bad.

I admire my Uncle Joe for many reasons, but one of the most important reasons is the fact that he was always there for me and never let me down. My Uncle Joe had to be one of the best police officers in New York State history, and they will never be the same without him. He had dignity and great pride in doing the right thing. As you can tell from what I write about my Uncle Joe, he has made a positive impact on my life and I will miss him very much. May you rest in peace Uncle Joe. I love you and miss you more than you will ever know.

Dear Uncle Joe,

I miss you! It has been three years on Friday since you were here with us. It's been very hard, every family get-together, there is a missing piece. That piece is you. I wish you were back with us so you could enjoy the stuff we used to do. Lake George trips, hunting, and get-togethers and so much more of what we used to do! I wish I could go back and know what was going to happen so I could have done more with you or maybe even changed the way things happened completely. I am glad that I was able to know you for as long as I was able to know you, I just wish you could still be here with us today.

Love you forever and always, Elliott or 'Clown'

Dear Uncle Joe,

Just writing your name makes me tear up. There are so many things that I miss about you. You were a great caring and loving uncle. You always put a smile on everyone's face. Most importantly- You were my God Father and I looked up to you for many things. I wish that you were still here with me and the rest of the family today, so we could have more and more memories together. It seems like just yesterday you were at my house and you were playing horse shoes out back with Uncle Jim, Grandpa, and Uncle Mike. We would do anything to have you back here with us today. You won't be able to see me graduate from high school or from college. I wish Joey and Dasia would have been able to call you their uncle. They would have loved you. I wish I could have been there the day you died, I would have done anything to still have you here with me and the rest of the family today! I miss you more than anything in the world Uncle Joe. I love you Uncle Joe! I wish I could have just one more day with you! I just want one more time to be able to give you a hug and tell you that I love you. I wouldn't have wanted anyone else to have been my God Father!

I love you Uncle Joe! More than anything else!

Love, Lizzy Austin

This poem was written by a family friend (Bonnylyn Buckley)
and read at Joe's funeral.

JOEY BANISH

I've loved Joey Banish
Since he was just a kid
Now, we have talked and we have laughed
And boy, I've picked on him

Even as a teenager
He was courteous and kind
One of the finest lads
You could ever find

Oh, he could be silly
But he was also smart
And he was the kind of kid
That wrapped around your heart

First a sweet young gentle boy
Then a grown up friend
Even when we didn't meet
For days or years on end

I know some troops who've worked with him
(And one of them is mine)
And all of their memories
Are positive and kind

'Cause when that young man came to work
He was set to go
He walked in with that special smile
That we'd all come to know

And it seems he did quite well
They could really work with him
That's a talent few folks have
A compliment to him!

He was such a human man
His attitude was great
And human ness is such a part
Of our eternal fate

So, let's remember this neat man
With reverence and joy
And all those social qualities
That came from that sweet boy

Please stand up to honor him
For God and man to see
Remember him with joy and love
Grant him peace and harmony*
*Eternal Calm

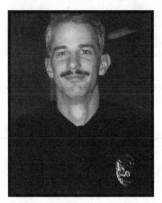

JAMES CROSS
January 21, 1968—March 24, 2008
Biography by Kerry Cross (Brother)

James Michael Cross was born in Durham, North Carolina on January 21, 1968 to James Marion Cross and Linda Pruitt Cross. Growing up, Michael enjoyed playing baseball and basketball for area little league teams. He loved to water ski and spent many summers at Kerr Lake with the family enjoying water sports. Michael joined the Boy Scouts at a young age and participated in many activities. Michael attended Northern Durham High School where he made good grades and the honor roll. He began working at Sears before he graduated and worked his way up to a manager's position. While holding that position, Michael met his first wife, Teresa. After graduating from high school, Michael and Teresa married and had two beautiful children. Michael loved to spend time with his children, taking them to the park and the zoo. Michael eventually applied for a job in security at Sears and began working in Loss Prevention where he met several of his future friends who worked for the police department.

Michael's little brother, Kerry, loved to annoy him at every chance he got. One summer when the boys were younger, Michael had a girlfriend over to the house and he threatened to beat the tar out of Kerry if he embarrassed him. Being the brat that Kerry was, he had to take Michael up on his dare. When Michael and his girlfriend settled into the TV room for quiet time alone, Kerry set the plot. Before being kicked out of the TV room, Kerry had opened the curtains. He then went outside and peered through the window. At the right moment, just when Michael was going to lay the first kiss on his girlfriend, Kerry began shouting and banging on the window. Michael was off the couch and out the front door before Kerry could escape. As Kerry puts it, time had come to pay the piper.

Mike was very ingenious. He was often placed in charge of his little brother while mom ran errands and dad was at work. Mike was none too happy with that assignment because the neighborhood kids had planned a football game. Michael had convinced the kids to play in his yard so he could be home with Kerry (his little brother). Then he came up with the grand idea. The idea was that if he could place Kerry in an area where he could not get in trouble, he would have nothing to worry about. So, Michael tricked his brother into a little game. That game was to handcuff his little brother to the bed post in his bedroom so he couldn't go anywhere or get in any trouble while he played football. As Kerry put it "A great ide... for Michael." Michael taught his little brother a lot about using his imagination and resources.

Growing up, Michael wore his heart on his sleeve. He enjoyed his friends and loved to make people laugh. If he felt like he had hurt someone or if someone did something to hurt him, intentional or not, it made him upset. Michael liked to be accepted and make new friends. He sometimes stood out among friends and strangers with his sense of humor. Michael never hesitated to help others out, strangers as well as friends.

He always jumped at the chance to make a new friend and would always lend a hand if they needed it. He spent his spare time assembling model cars, planes, and space ships. Michael enjoyed playing basketball with friends at church and participated in youth church programs. Every chance he got,

Michael would attend Durham Bulls baseball games with friends, family and his kids.

He became interested in law enforcement while participating in the Boy Scouts in a program much like the Explorer Program of today. From those days of interest, he knew he was going to be a police officer. Michael grew up watching 70's and 80's television police shows like SWAT, Adam 12, and COPS. Some of his other favorite TV shows were Star Trek and M*A*S*H.

Michael pursued his interest in law enforcement and eventually applied for the Durham Police Department. He was accepted and hired on January 9, 1995. Michael attended the Durham Police Academy and was sworn in on May 12, 1995. Michael was very proud of his accomplishments and worked very hard to achieve his goals in the police department. On April 23, 1997 he began working within the police department as a Field Training Officer. On May 4, 1998 he received recognition for good conduct and was promoted to the position of Corporal on July 1, 1999.

Michael did some of his patrol work on a bike and worked closely with local citizens as he worked in the Community Policing Program. He resigned from the Durham Police Department on October 20, 2004.

Michael got divorced and remarried towards the end of his career with the police department. In his second marriage he had another beautiful child. Michael's wife Katie, received a job offer in Florida so they packed up the family and moved there. Michael wanted to stay away from police work for a while so he worked several jobs outside of the law enforcement profession. Eventually he found a job in security at a large, local firm.

Michael began to experience some significant personal issues in his life. He became separated from his second wife and fell into a major depression. After several months of mental pain, Michael took his own life with his service weapon which he had purchased from his police department.

James Michael Cross, an American hero, died at his own hand on March 24, 2008. The last contact he had with his children was also on that date.

Letter to Michael from Kerry (Brother)

Dear Bro,

Where do I start? You are sorely missed by so many people. It has been two years and there is still so much pain, anger, and sadness. I am not going to ask why because I think we all know why and that the question can never be fully answered. You lost focus for a short amount of time and took so much away from us leaving a sense of loss that will last forever. Three children will never know their father and the man he could have been. A father will never be able to heal the wounds that he felt he caused and a brother will always live with the pain of thinking he had done good.

Growing up, we never really got along too well. You were the older, mature, career oriented brother and I was the younger, immature brat who ruined your dates and stayed on your nerves every chance I got. You had a totally different set of friends and we always had different goals. But when you were hurting, I hurt. When you got into a fight with neighbor kids, I got angry. Remember when you got in a fight and your little brother came out with a bat swinging? You got so mad at me for coming to save the day. I didn't say a word because I knew you appreciated it but you were embarrassed.

I remember when you first learned to water ski slalom. I wanted so badly, to be like you. I wanted to ski like you and be like my big brother. Of course, I would never tell you that, because it just would not have been cool. Instead I played it down and acted like it was no big deal.

When I got in trouble at work, the same place you worked, I felt horrible. The only real thought I had was that I had disappointed my big brother and you would hate me forever. You let me know that was not the case. I don't think I ever told you but I was so sorry.

We never really hung out together growing up and we grew even farther apart as we grew older. You married, had kids and moved away. I finally graduated from high school and moved to another county to go to school. We would be together mostly during holidays and special events. I came home to see my niece and nephew and spend some time with the family.

I remember when you had your first child, my niece. I will never forget that I was the first one you wanted to come back in the hospital room to hold her. Man, that was cool. I could just see the pride in your eyes. You were glowing. Then came the birth of your son. You were so ready to show him how to "be a man," teach him how to play basketball, and send him off to the big leagues... every hope of a father.

I will always remember the day you graduated from the police academy. I was so proud seeing you walk down the aisle with your uniform on.

I used to tell everyone that my brother was a police officer in one of the most violent cities around. It was a huge pride thing to know that you could do that and perform your job so well.

Then there was Las Vegas. When you asked if I wanted to go to the "Sin City" with you for a couple of days, I wasn't quite sure. What would we talk about? What would we do? We were two totally different people. I am so glad I went! We had a really good time and bonded in a way that we needed to do for many years. Even though we came back broke and had nothing to show for going, there were a lot of positives in the trip.

When things became bad in your life and you turned to your

little brother, we were talking every day, several times a day. I could tell that you were hurting and needed someone to talk to. I tried so hard to give advice, options, and any help I knew of.

The night that you told me you could not take it any more, I immediately went to you. I quit my life, bought a plane ticket, and got to you as quickly as I could. This is the time I will cherish forever. We spent four days talking, laughing, and sharing stories of our childhood. You told me how you were jealous of me and the things I had accomplished. I told you how proud I was of that you were my brother. We took long walks and drives and just recapped our lives. The day I left to return home, I truly thought we had worked through a lot together and you would be okay. You were making efforts to heal old wounds and make things better in your life.

I should have seen the blinds when you asked for my address. When you said "I lost your address and need it for my address book." Shortly after that I received your text that said "Love ya bro." My heart sank but I did not want to believe this was a bad sign. I replied "I love you too bro?" Did you ever see that? How did you feel?

The next day I could not get in touch with you. You would not answer my text messages or phone calls. I called someone and asked that they go to your house and check on you. Your truck was there but you were not answering the door. Hell began to play on me. The police were called and I waited for what seemed like forever to hear something. I paced back and forth in the house and just sat on the floor waiting. Waiting to hear something.

When the call finally came, the first thing out of the other person's mouth was "I am sorry." I broke, became confused, angry, and in total disbelief. I grabbed my car keys and headed to daddy's house. I made the one hour drive in 30 minutes. I had to get to him and your children before anyone else told them. When I told daddy what had happened, the sadness and disbelief were almost too much but I still had to get to the children. Daddy and I rushed over to the kid's house, hardly speaking a word to each other. I felt as if my feet were in concrete as I walked up to their doorstep. I had to push myself to that door. When I told them their father was dead, you could feel the pain in the air. The silence was so uncomfortable as everyone sat in confusion. I was mad that I had to tell them what you had done but I knew it was I who needed to tell them.

If you had only known the pain we would all have to endure, even two years later, would you still have done it? If you could have seen the attendance at your funeral, the support and people who approached me and said they enjoyed working with you. It didn't feel real that I would be burying my brother.

I received your letter in the days following the funeral. That is why you wanted my address. You wanted to send a letter to me because you had plans. How could I have not seen this coming? I thought everything was going well. The cliché that suicide is a permanent answer to a temporary problem plays true. We could have worked through this Michael. You could have seen your daughter graduate from high school and go on to college. If you would have just held on.

I wanted to fix the pain for you and was willing to help in any way I could. I wanted to help you get back on track because, in the end, I love you Bro.

Kerry

Letter to Mike from his dad

Michael,

I love you more than you could ever know, but the act of taking your own life is devastating. You have hurt and saddened all your family and friends, to the point of anger and disappointment.

You had family and friends who loved you, and would have done anything they could to help you. You have missed your children growing up and graduating from school, getting married and having future grandchildren. The tears and hurt will always be there, but my love for you will never end. There is never a day that goes by that I don't think about you. God, family and friends were there to help in any way possible. You are missed and will never be forgotten.

Love,
    Dad

Letter from Teresa (Former wife)

Mike,

It only seems right that I write this letter today, December 20th because it was this day 24 years ago that we were married. That day was the start of dreams we had for ourselves. I miss those days. I miss when we would just have simple nights of renting a good movie and just snuggling on the couch. I remember the conversations we would have about what our children would be like and how proud you were when they both were born. You had Amber's whole name picked out a year before we knew we were expecting. Thank God she was a girl! Then Jordan came along. You had a son to carry your name now. We felt our family was complete. Then hearing you made it into the police academy, I was so proud of you! This was your dream since you were little and now it looked as though all of your dreams came true. I remember the day you came home from the academy feeling you could not do it. I knew you could. You made it through that tough period to graduation.

Your job was never easy but I was always so proud of you, even when you brought work home. Even though our marriage did not last through it, I still always loved you. I should have told you that the last time you called pleading for forgiveness. I felt your pain as you talked and told me how you now understand the pain you had put the children and me through. Now that I look back on that conversation, I see that you were not only asking for my forgiveness but also saying good-bye.

We miss you and what should have been. I do not think less of you. I know you were hurting. The children still ask why.

Sometimes I do too, even though I know the answer. Amber wanted her father at her graduation. I knew you were there. Did you hear my prayers the night before? I told you that you were needed there. We were to experience this together. This was our first-born. Amber wanted to know why you couldn't have waited. Then maybe you would have changed your mind if you had. I knew you were there though. I remember walking to the building at Duke University and I felt your presence.

At first I didn't know what it was. Then after stopping several times to see who was walking beside me and seeing no one, it hit me. That presence I felt beside me was you. I felt as though I could reach out and grab your hand. I knew then that you did not desert us. Not spiritually. I know you will always be with us. One day I know that I will see you again in heaven. Until then, know we miss you dearly and all of the life experiences that we should be sharing with you.

You are always in my heart,
Teresa

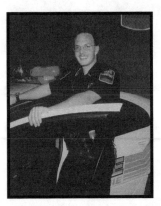

ERIC CHARLES FEIFER
December 12, 1976—January 6, 2006
Biography by Katie Moreno

Early December 1976, in a small southern Wisconsin town, Eric Feifer was born. A beautiful, brown haired, brown eyed baby boy. Four years later he became a big brother to a baby sister; it seemed he was destined for the role of protector. Around the time Eric was five years old, his mother remarried and he gained a step brother and sister, all of whom would remain best friends throughout his life. It was clear from an early age , Eric possessed a compassionate and nurturing spirit, that with time, would play a prominent role in his personality. His life was not one of ease and privilege however, it was how he turned any disadvantage into something positive that made him so exceptional.

Like most kids growing up where money is a constant struggle and home was often moved around, life could feel unfair and difficult. In his young years, life had given him some heavy burdens to carry, but he didn't complain. Even though there must have been pain, disappointment, and insecurity, he didn't surrender to it or blame anyone. He understood that he had a choice, a choice to take a different path, one that could make him happy and that's exactly what he set out to do.

Eric moved out on his own at the age of seventeen. He worked full time jobs to support himself while attending college. He knew what he wanted and was willing to work hard to get it. It wasn't long before he graduated and he set his attentions to putting all the pieces in place.

Throughout the next couple of years, Eric worked his way up through small time security gigs and eventually, in 2001, became a police officer with a small village police department. He loved his job and was dedicated. He also just so happened to be very good at it. The image of the iconic police officer, strong, fearless and caring was everything that Eric was. He made it seem effortless. There are those people you meet in life who seem to define their roles and set standards others strive to meet. Professionally, there wasn't a better fit for him.

There could be a million things written about what a charitable person Eric was.

Reaching into his own pocket so that a homeless man could get a hot meal and then giving him a ride to get it. Taking the time to console a scared little girl who just witnessed a brutal fight between her parents so she would know she wasn't alone. Simply lending an ear to someone who needed one. He never asked for recognition for any of this, that wasn't why he did it. There was never an agenda or expectation of reward. He did these things because that's who he was. He understood what fear was, how hunger felt, and the pain and loneliness of disappointment. He helped people because somehow, it righted those wrongs for himself.

In 2002 Eric met and fell in love with someone who was lucky enough to recognize him for the beautiful person he was. They started building a life together and things couldn't have been more perfect. A wedding was planned, a house was bought, so many dreams, so many possibilities. His life of course, wouldn't be complete without little creatures he could care for; two puppies, Honey and Mia and two cats, Tazzy and Vinnie. It was a mad house at times but always a warm one. This house became the place to celebrate holidays and birthdays or just a gathering place for friends and family; there was a lot of love in Eric's home.

People liked Eric for many reasons but probably the most apparent was his incredible sense of humor. He was the funny guy. He had a quick wit and could always make you laugh. He had a collection of obscure celebrity impressions, most of which were eerily good. He was serious when he needed to be, but he had a knack for finding the humor in everything. Much of his charm came from the most ridiculous things he would come up with. Strange nonsensical sayings were much a part of that. One in particular sticks out as a good example. One time he said "I just feel like a three legged dog guarding the farm." The situation to which he was referring is unclear but it sure didn't involve dogs or farms. Eric had millions of these, some making even less sense.

Another well known Eric-ism was how extremely particular he was about being organized. Organized probably isn't the right word to use—this was a true skill. Perhaps a strange thing to be known for but this was one of those "You had to be there" things, to truly understand. Even the labels had labels.

In his world, everything had its place. As a result, he had to suffer from time to time because sometimes, it was just too much temptation not to add a little chaos to all that order and move everything around (per his fiancé, Katie). Eric was good natured about it; of course he immediately had to move everything back. It certainly wasn't a bad compulsion to have; at least he never lost anything.

Eric never left a room without letting the people in it know he loved them. When he hugged you, you felt it was real. There was no performance behind it. He lived simply, gratefully, and piously.

To himself, it may have seemed unremarkable, but to those he touched, it was far from ordinary. We have all met people in our lives where we instantly recognize something different or special about them. Something deeper, wiser, it's an unavoidable attraction. As if they know things the rest of us don't. Eric set his standards high for himself but he never judged or criticized, he just accepted everyone as they were. He made people want to be better because of it. He probably didn't even realize that. That's why everyone loved Eric Feifer.

Eric Charles Feifer, an American Hero, died at his own hand on Friday, January 6, 2006.

Letter from Katie Moreno (Fiancé)

Eric,

It's been a long time since we talked... I miss you. No matter how much time goes by, this never gets any easier. There is so much I want to say to you that I don't know where to start. So many things have changed since you left that it's hard to recognize this world sometimes.

I feel like I need to make sure you don't miss out on anything. I take little mental notes, a funny joke I heard or something crazy that happened at work. I imagine that you would laugh but I don't ever really tell you these things. I just end up feeling foolish; All these little things don't matter. After all, there's really only one thing that I need you to know, "I love you."

Sometimes I think back to all the things we've done., We had some pretty good adventures. It's hard to imagine those are the only memories I will ever get to have of you. We can never make more. No more laughs, no more talks, no more completely senseless road trips to nowhere just for the heck of it. I miss all of it. Although I will cherish what I have, it will never be the same. I can't put my arms around a memory.

It's getting better but God knows I still struggle with all this. Feeling like I've been cursed one day then defeated the next. Five years later and I'm still a complete mess. Perhaps that's normal, I'm not sure. It's hard not to be resentful and some days I wish I could just forget you. Don't worry though, it's all temporary and I don't mean it. Tomorrow I'll remember how lucky I had been to know you, even if only for that short time.

I realize we all make decisions in life, sometimes at the

expense of others, unintentionally causing pain we are sorry for later. I know you did what you felt you had to do and regardless of how much it hurts, I know you didn't intend for it to be this way.

You will always be my best friend and I will always be thankful for every minute I got to spend with you.

I love you Eric,
     Katie

Letter to Eric from his sister

E,

We waited for you to come home that night. Four years later, we continue to. Since that moment, time has frozen in a cycle of memory and past tenses. That ephemeral mark on the past has immovably ruptured the possibility of the present and the future. Traumatic moments, quickly lose the signifier of "short," and instead, burrow themselves with a driving momentum, into every hour, minute, day, and month that follows.

Waiting for someone who will never return, is not the same as pining. It's not the feeling of a lovelorn heart in a state of longing. In those situations, a viable hope for a reunion remains. The death of a loved one, on the contrary, is a silence. The unexpected loss is an arresting disquietude. There is nothing peaceful, nor healing about this silence. These are not moments to glean clarity from the tranquil mind. "The Year of Magical Thinking," has turned into five for me.

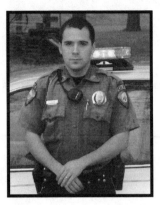

BRIAN MATHEW RESSER
January 18, 1986 — June 23, 2009
Biography by his mother

Brian Mathew Resser was born January 18th, 1986 at the Memorial Hospital in Manhattan, Kansas.

Brian was such a happy little boy who always had a mischievous smile on his face. He was always on the go and wouldn't even stop long enough to take a nap; he would fall asleep in his high chair at the evening meal. When he ran, it was like he bounced with each step he took. Brian's hair turned very blonde when he was two years old and his parents were teased constantly about how and where Brian got his blonde hair. Brian had a great sense of humor. He loved a good joke and could even play a few on people... he enjoyed teasing.

Brian went out for both football and track in middle school. In track, he received medals for nearly every running event he participated in. Brian competed in track all the way through high school (until an ankle injury sidelined him his senior year). His specialty was the 400m and the 4X400m relay. Twice during his high school year Brian competed at the State level and he earned a medal for both of his categories his first year of State level competition. He was also in the high school marching band as a percussionist.

One of the things Brian enjoyed the most was hanging out with his brothers. They loved to hunt and fish together. Brian enjoyed family and friends and especially loved get-togethers when he and his brothers and sisters played Wii or X-Box. Even as an adult, Brian was as energetic as when he was as a little boy—he was always on the move. He never just sat at home. He enjoyed watching television shows like *The Simpsons* and *Family Guy*. Brian kept in touch with everybody and liked to send text messages. He sent a text to his parents nearly every day.

Brian loved cars and at the time of his death he was in the process of restoring a 1978 Trans Am. Brian and his dad spent many hours working on cars together ever since he was a kid. Brian loved to buy and trade cars. His last collection included a 1967 Camaro and a 1968 Trans Am.

Brian was a loyal Green Bay fan and enjoyed watching Bret Favre. Brian's parents bought him tickets to the NFL game (Kansas City Chiefs vs. Green Bay Packers) when they came to Kansas City. Brian was completely excited and sent texts and pictures to his parents while he watched the game.

Brian graduated from Wamego High School with the class of 2005. After graduation, he attended Barton College for auto mechanics (more confirmation of his love for cars).

In 2007 Brian was hired by Herington Police Department and on November 21, 2008 Brian completed his law enforcement training in Hutchinson, Kansas and became a police officer with Herington Police Department. Brian was a member of the First Baptist Church Herington and on July 9, 2008 he married JoLynn Williams at that very church. He has two beautiful children, Jadyn Hagen and Julian Mathew Resser.

Brian loved being a police officer and eventually was hired by Wabaunsee Sheriff's Office. At the time of his death, Brian worked for Wabaunsee County Sheriff's Office and part time at the Herington Police Department.

On June 23, 2009, Brian Mathew Resser, an American Hero, died at his own hand as he sat in his car in Herington, Kansas

Letter to Brian from JoLynn Resser (Wife)

Brian and I met in April of 2008, he was handsome and I was interested. We had our first date that May...We went bowling and had lunch at Chili's. I had a great time getting to know him better. On July 9, 2008 we married. I was expecting and in love. Brian went to the police academy that August and was gone every week for three months. When our son was born, Brian and I named him Julian Matthew. It was one of the best days of my life. Brian seemed so happy but he became distant when he changed jobs from our small town to a larger area where he became a deputy sheriff. I loved and still love Brian so much and every day I wonder how I am going to tell our son why this happened to us....why his daddy won't be there for his first day of school, his baseball games, his graduation, or his wedding.

Brian,

I have questioned every day, what happened to you, how it got to this point, and how you left all the people who loved you the most. I know these questions will never be answered. I don't know the exact reasons why you chose to take your life but I wish every day you would've seen that the good outweighs the bad. We have a beautiful son who someday will go through the same things we all have gone through. He will still have to grieve for you and I am unsure of how to help. You also have a daughter who will someday ask her mother why she doesn't have her father to walk her down the aisle. I thank God every day that Julian will have his sister Jadyn, to grow up with and to share his feelings and thoughts with...They already have a great relationship.

I want to tell you how much I love you and still think of you every day and read the letters you wrote to me. I talk out loud to you and I see your pictures every day. We miss you so much. Julian tells me, when he sees a picture of you, "That's my Daddy". It is amazing! I just wish you were to be with him, to watch him grow and evolve into the amazing little person he is. I don't know how you felt that day but I replay it over and remember the fear and sorrow in your voice. I know you didn't want to do it but you felt you had no other choice. The first thing you said to me that night was "Tell Julian that I love him and that this had nothing to do with him." The last thing you told me was "I love you and I am so sorry." When the phone went dead that night, a piece of me died with it. I wonder every day what I could've said to prevent you from doing what you did. I want you here with Julian so bad and I know some day we will be at peace with what happened. I'm just not sure when that day will come. We love you very much Brian. You will never be forgotten.

Letter to Brian from his mother

Dear Brian,

We all loved you so much. A part of me died with you that morning. Our family will never be whole again. Every holiday, wedding, anniversary, birthday, and family event; there is a constant sadness that can never be lifted. I will never be truly happy again; your absence is always on my mind. The loss of a child is the absolute worst thing a parent can experience.

I am so sorry I feel like I failed you in some way. I would give anything to have you back again, to hear your voice, to give you a hug and tell you how much I love you again. I would have done anything for you; there was nothing I would not have done to help you. There is not a moment in a day that I don't think about you and miss you.

Your children will never know what a great young man you were. I will not get to see you play with them, or to help them through life. Every time I see a father with a child, I think of you and what your children will miss without you and what we will all miss, not having you in our lives.

Every night before I go to bed, I go outside, look up to the heavens and tell you that I love and miss you. My hope is that you are at peace and have the contentment that eluded you here on earth. I love and miss you so very much. I will till I take my last breath.

Love You, Mom

Letter to Brian from his father

Dear Brian,

I really feel like I should have done more stuff with you but I really thought that I would be taking time away from you that you would be spending with your family; you were so busy with your job and the time you were spending with Jason and Shawn.

The thing I wish you could have known was how many friends you really had and the time you will now never have with your kids watching them grow. I can see you in them every time I see them. How they look and how quick they are to understand how things work. They are very good with their hands, just like you were.

I feel like we really could have worked things out if we could have sat down and talked about it. I know I did not have the answer you wanted to hear but at least we could have tried something, anything. We would have found the answer, sooner or later.

The most important thing I would tell you is how much I love you and how much I miss you.

Love,
   Dad

Letter to Brian from Shawn

Dear Brian,

I know you are in a better place now that your heart is at rest. I don't know what drove you to it, but I just wanted to say I love you. Everywhere I go I see something or someone that reminds me of you. I know you are with God, for he told me at your funeral. You see, that day when the minister asked us all to pray for you, I asked God to give me a sign that you were with him. I asked him to show me a butterfly or something, just to let me know. When we went downstairs after the funeral, I looked up and on almost every crossbeam was a butterfly. I hadn't noticed them there before. On the way to the cemetery where you were to be buried, I was looking out the window and there was another one flying around for me to see. After it was all said and done and we all went home, I looked out the kitchen window only to see one more flying around mom's flowers. So, I know you are with God and have found peace.

I also know you were at Sarah's wedding. She told me that when she was setting up for her wedding, she asked you if you were going to be there. She had your picture on one of the chairs in the front row, and you knocked your picture over several times.

I just want you to know that I love you a lot and miss you a lot. But I know I'll be seeing you all over the place. I hope you will be there at our wedding to watch Jessica and I get married, and to share in our wonderful day together. I know I will see you around.

Love,
Shawn

Letter to Brian from Jason

Brian,

It has been a year and a half since you died, yet it feels like only yesterday. It's hard to explain the heartache that was caused by you leaving the way you did. Suicide is hard to deal with. I think it would have been easier to hear you had died in an accident. There would have been some kind of closure. But you took your own life, you made a choice to give up, to let go, leaving us behind to clean up the shattered lives.

We all knew you were going through hard times, but what we didn't know, is how much it was eating at you. You needed someone to talk to, someone to listen, and confide in, but you didn't want to tell anyone. Maybe because you thought you were going to be judged, or that we would think that you couldn't handle the problems that had been created. We all knew the day would come when you would have to deal with the problems that had been building for years. Life has a funny way of catching up with you. Life wasn't always fair with you either, it always seemed that you were always dealt a short hand. It was kind of your personality. You always seemed to make the most of it, but I knew that nothing ever turned out how you really wanted and it was eating at you.

One of the hardest things now is to see your kids. Jules looks so much like you. It almost kills me inside to see him. To see your child photos and see him is almost a perfect match. To know also, that he will never again see his dad, or get to know him, kills me. Also, your daughter; a father's daughter is hard to explain, they always have a close spot in a father's heart. To know that she will never remember you and that my children will never remember you hurts. Brian, you were so close to my daughter. I know that you loved her like your own. One of the saddest days I can remember happened only a few months ago when our photo of you fell off the TV stand and my daughter picked it up and asked who you were. She knew Shawn but not you. She was too young when you took your life, to remember your face now. After you two had been so close, she couldn't even remember your name.

Nothing has been the same since you left. Life got complicated with the family. Holidays bring sorrow, seeing your kids, and then thinking of how different it would be if you were still alive. I wish things were different. I wish you were still here.

I remember one of the last things you said to me before you left. We were hunting and you dreamed of when Jules and Tanner were old enough to join us. We were going to go on a hunting trip, just us and the boys. It was one of the few times I had really seen you happy. Knowing that I had a son on the way and that we would be doing stuff together for a long time made me happy.

You have missed a lot of stuff in your absence. Sarah got married and she just learned on her birthday this year, that she is pregnant. Shawn is engaged to be married this year also. You also missed your best friend's wedding. You will miss seeing all of Sarah's and Shawn's children grow up and you never got to see my boy. They will never get to know or even meet you Brian. It's not an easy thing to think about. I wish things were different. I think all of us do. We all miss you but I know you're watching out for me. I know you're watching out for all of us. We miss you a lot.

Jason

Letter to Brian Resser from John Pritchard (Chief of Police)

Dear Brian,

Not a day goes by at the Herington Police Department that we don't think about you and mourn your death. Your absence has created a huge void in our lives. We had seen you mature into a fine young officer and many of us had developed a close personal friendship with you. I was honored to be the best man at your wedding and enjoyed getting to know you and your family. Officer Eugene Ray III was looking forward to you being the best man at his wedding and after your death, he left the best man position unfilled.

You told me that law enforcement was the best career that you had ever had and how much you enjoyed it. You had the potential to do great things with your life and even though your life ended at the age of 23 you had already impacted many people in many positive ways. You were a private person who wanted to handle his own problems but you felt that you had lost control of your personal life. As a law enforcement officer, that was particularly frustrating to you because you were used to being in control and solving other people's problems but you couldn't solve your own.

We understand that the sadness and depression you were experiencing was more than you felt you could bear and we have not judged you. Rather, we have chosen to remember you for the person who you really were and for all the positive contributions that you made during your lifetime. We will not let one regrettable act erase all the good things you did with your life. Law enforcement officers are human too and we all face the same problems and difficulties as other people.

The night that you died, you made it clear that you had no intention of hurting anyone other than yourself. But your decision did hurt others because it caused pain to all the people who cared about you and that pain will never go away. You were well respected in the community and many people came forward with stories after you died of how you had touched their lives by caring and talking with them, on and off duty.

Being buried in your uniform was the highest honor we could give to you and your funeral was well attended. During the funeral procession on I-70, a rural Herington couple who were traveling home on motorcycle saw the three police cars escorting the hearse and funeral procession. They realized it was you and pulled over to the shoulder of the highway and stood next to their motorcycles as the procession passed. HPD placed a memorial in the newspaper and we placed a memorial plaque[1] in the lobby of the police department to preserve your memory. The phrase at the bottom of the plaque reads, *"You made a difference of the lives of others."*

Brian, you touched the lives of everyone who knew you and you will never be forgotten. Our prayer is that you have found the peace in the next world that had eluded you in this one, and that your friends and family may continue to find peace and healing in their lives as well. Rest in peace.

Your friend,
John Pritchard
Chief of Police

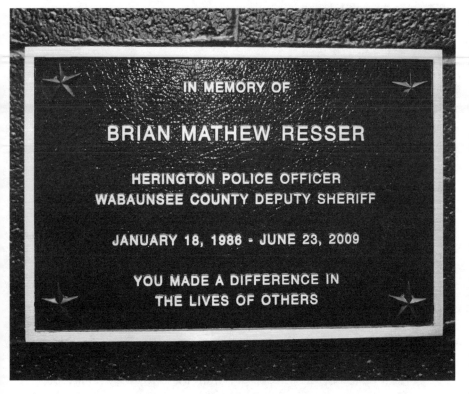

*1-Photograph of the plaque displayed in the Herington Police Department
lobby in Herington, Kansas.

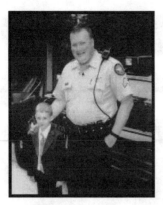

TIMOTHY B. THACKER
October 9, 1966—February 28, 2008
Biography by Pamela F. Thacker (Wife)

They sing in Oklahoma... "OKLA-OKLA-OKLA-OKLA-OKLA-OKLA... We know we belong to the land, and the land we belong to is grand!" Well, That certainly was the case in the life of Oklahoman, Timothy Brian Thacker, who was brought into this world, compliments of a military doctor by the handy use of forceps at Fort Sill Oklahoma on October 9, 1966. He weighed in at 8lbs 3 oz. and resided on base with his mother, Lois Harrison Thacker and father, Emmett Marvin Thacker who was an infantryman in the good old United States Army during the Vietnam era. In the early years, Tim loved Winnie The Pooh (one of his favorite childhood toys) and hated to get his hands dirty.

After his father was discharged from the army they returned to Georgia and family was a huge part of his upbringing. There were many get-togethers with cousins and he never missed a Mother Thacker Christmas Party with his relatives. His grandmother, Idabelle Thacker would giggle while telling of how he would sit up and flip through the phone book for hours at times as a young boy. G.I. Joe was another favorite past time and Tim had quite a collection, often entertaining "War Play" with neighborhood friends. Growing up, he was an active young man who resided in the Stone Mountain area and was baptized at Rolling Hills Baptist Church. The family decided to build a home in 1979 on Round Ridge Road in Loganville, Georgia.

Tim began school at Loganville Middle and his family

attended Victory Baptist Church, along with neighborhood friend Spencer Pratt, often known as his accomplice in good clean mischief. His cousin Jeff Smith would visit often and if there was a bb gun involved, it was bad news. They once even shot a bird off the power line. Right as Jeff pulled the trigger, the neighbor lady screamed out "Don't shoot my..." It was too late. They had no idea of course it was her pet and they took off running through the woods back to the house. He played recreation baseball and football but was a lean man who ended up preferring baseball. In high school, Tim Thacker was the quiet one who never claimed any certain social group. He was an average teenager who worked part time with a local heating and air company.

He attended church weekly with his mother and sister and often helped teach Sunday School. He loved John Wayne and sported a green beret almost daily his senior year. He had a strong desire to serve his country in combat. He was one heck of a runner, quick on his feet, and often was the pinch runner of the high school Red Devil baseball team to ensure home plate was passed and another run went up on the scoreboard. A few of his favorite teachers included Ms. Diane Alexander, his delightfully difficult English teacher and Ms. Gina Green Luck, his French teacher who was also in the military guard.

Interestingly, he did not speak a lick of French but would often write his "High School Sweetheart" love letters in the language that she would have to decipher to understand. He loved Mr. Mance Mapp, who was a very stern disciplinarian with a very large paddle he titled "The Enforcer" (and still has it to this day).

Tim loved to push buttons a little, such as "Taking baby steps off the school bus" or entertaining them with an occasional "Full Moon." Tim also started the "Camo fad" and should've added the title, Camo Fashion Designer behind his name as this fad continues to live on through the years. If there was a different pattern made, he had one of each green/tan it didn't matter, with a field jacket to match. After graduation he worked as a glazier for Peach state Glass Company and found excitement in repelling from high-rise buildings doing specialty glass work. The next few years were full of events such as more homecoming dances, football games, proms, etc. as he continued to date waiting for the love of his life to graduate. The couple enjoyed outdoor activities together such as swimming, long walks, repelling, and target shooting. Both Tim and his girlfriend loved softball.

In August of 1987, on a very hot day, the 23rd, he made Pamela Faye Rogers his wife. After dating almost four years, the couple established a life together in Loganville, Georgia. They were members of Corinth Christian Church. Captain Johnny Smith, who often worked Loganville High School extra-curricular events, continued to remind Tim that Walton County was in need of officers. The idea was thrown around many times but taking the job would have meant an $8.00 per hour pay cut. In January of 1988, Tim began Jailer school (he gave in). Pam supported Tim's dream of serving his community and they both felt the pay cut, although substantial, would allow Tim to perform more meaningful work.

He had many boring days early on as there was not much crime back then, however, just months after he started with Walton County, he was sent back to Northeast Georgia Police Academy in Athens for the position of Deputy Sheriff. He was also part of the Governor's Drug Task Force in which a helicopter flight crew would search for local grow sights and when located, the team would disassemble the sight. Road patrol offered a variety of shift work, as well as a variety of tasks performed during that shift.

Tim often worked the evening shift, 11:00 pm to 7:00 a.m. and had a pivotal moment around the first of the year early in 1990, just weeks before his child was born. When Tim arrived home that morning, Pam looked out the window to find every single part of his patrol car dented and almost every window broken... it was a startling sight. Tim Shared with Pam that he was so close to resigning because he could not depend on his backup. Upon having to shut down an out of control party in a bad neighborhood , he phoned for back up. He had two other similar calls that night, (in regards to the same address) and radio was notified to send backup ASAP.

Unfortunately, his back up did not show up. In the process of working the call, he was on edge because the attendees were very intoxicated and unpredictable. The owner of the home was arrested by Tim but not so easily. You see, the locals there were not so happy about the party being shut down and a group of about 15+ surrounded the patrol car and began rocking it. Another 5-10 began hurling very large landscaping rocks repeatedly, hitting and denting the patrol car. Deputy Thacker, in an attempt to leave the premises, found himself in a position alone with a group of approximately 40+ individuals who were not pleased with the arrest. Without notice "Crash!"—the back window was busted in and a rock entered the car and struck the passenger who had been arrested. Broken glass was everywhere and Deputy Thacker took the PA and said "You have 3 seconds to move from the front of the car." One, two, and on three he mashed the accelerator and got out of there as fast as he could. It was a dangerous moment that left him wondering "Why am I doing this?" Well, it certainly wasn't for the money or the safety. He actually considered leaving the force that night as becoming a father was first and foremost on his mind.

And, he found himself thinking, "I could've lost my life tonight and never had the opportunity to hold my own child." On the force, the guys are taught to suck it up and like the military, just drive on! That's exactly what Tim did. Weeks later, May 18, 1990, Kristian Audrianna Thacker was born after a night of wiffle ball at church. Yes, Tim and Pam played wiffle ball with the Wednesday 5th and 6th grade class they taught at church. Tim was an excellent labor coach who had been trained in the Bradley Method® of child birth. Tim was even trained on how to help deliver his own child in the event his help was needed. He was dedicated and prepared and for twenty-two hours of back labor he performed heroically: he loved, he rubbed, he encouraged... he did everything necessary to help welcome his daughter into the world without unnecessary drugs and intervention. Finally, his hard work had paid off. Their daughter was born drug free and could not have been more perfect. It was a teamwork effort that paid off big.

The couple enjoyed the experience they later went and were trained to be a teaching couple of the Bradley Method® and yes, Tim remained a member of the police department and a full time father. The couple had made the decision to keep their children out of day care. Tim watched Kristian from 7:30 a.m. till around 2:00 p.m. and although the couple did not see much of each other during the week, they believed their parental sacrifices were worth all the trouble.

Then, another late night/early morning, Tim found himself rolling up on a fire scene. It appeared a car had left the roadway and struck a concrete ravine. It was fully engulfed in flames and there was absolutely nothing Deputy Thacker could do except call for fire dispatch and watch. The horrific images he expressed to his wife the next day would haunt him in his mind for weeks to come.

Continually, he could see the young lady through the driver's window, on fire, over and over, banging on the glass trying to get out.

There were quiet nights as well when the officers could check in on local business owners and simply catch up on things. Tim enjoyed interacting with the community in that fashion. He would often speak to the young children at vacation bible school events. He enjoyed sharing his career and allowing the children to check out the cool stuff in the car, etc. Those were proud moments for Tim Thacker.

In the years following, Tim would work his way up the ranks to sergeant and any high ranking officer would tell you that Tim was excellent at the Oral Boards (a Promotional Interview). There seemed to be no question that Tim did not know the answer to. He would study the County Manual and was always improving his knowledge with one continuing education class after another. He enjoyed the vast array of continuing education courses offered and available to him and he far exceeded the yearly requirements for training.

Tim was a very principled man who took pride in his position. But off duty, he was a jokester. He loved doing silly stuff to make people laugh. He enjoyed dumb movies such as *Dumb and Dumber* and *Super Troopers*. However, when it came to work, Deputy Thacker took an oath to enforce the law equally, fairly, and without prejudice and he did not discriminate against anyone. Deputy Thacker even locked his own father up for a DUI after warning him not to get behind the wheel. The department had a lot of laughs with that one.

Tim Thacker loved his family and had a deep appreciation of tough love. On May 19, 1992, his second daughter, Jocelyn Victoria Thacker, was born after the couple climbed Stone Mountain. Tired but full of laughter, they headed up to the hospital. Again, with Tim's excellent coaching, another daughter was born drug and intervention free. His love for fatherhood gleamed across his face. He remained at home watching his two year old and newborn daughter and he loved it! His daughters were both Daddy's Little Girls. He had given up the SWAT Team and his full time job as *Deputy* but considered his job as full time father to be much more rewarding. Happily, he enjoyed his time at home, loving his girls daily and teaching them necessary life lessons. He loved reading books to his girls and just laughing and playing with them. His "Mr. Mom" experience was one of the happiest times of his life.

In 1994, Tim returned to his beloved job but this time, it was serving Dekalb County Sheriff's Department as a Jailor. He seemed to enjoy the work most days but with 4800 inmates, the job had its challenges.

In 1996 his father was diagnosed with a terminal illness and Tim returned to Walton County for their twelve hour work shifts which allowed him to assist his mother in caring for his father. Tim began to work his way back up the ladder and regained his title of sergeant. Tim was on the Walton County Color Guard and took pride in their brotherhood. In 1997, Tim was left grieving, often feeling confused about why he had to lose his father. His dad was only 52 years old and passed at the University of

Birmingham Hospital, awaiting a lung transplant. He missed his father and the relationship and closeness they had developed while his dad was ill.

After his father's death, Tim's urge to serve his country was amplified. His family encouraged him to go for it and in September of 2000, he entered Fort Benning as an infantryman in training, just like his father had (only Tim started at an older age). Tim, being older than most of his Drill Instructors, was dubbed, "Moses." The family got a kick out of this and as far as they know, Tim still holds the record as the oldest and fastest at disassembling and assembling the M-14 rifle. He had no problem completing the physical requirements at 35 because he had prepared in advance, but following a fall which rendered him unable to run, the military doctors wanted to perform surgery on his knee. Financially at the time, this was not an option. An MRI later revealed unrepairable, permanent damage to the cartilage behind his knee cap. Tim was grateful for the opportunity to serve in the military, however his injury brought that career to an end.

Tim once again served his community through the Walton County Sheriff's Office. He and his wife coached Special Olympics at Loganville High and brought back several Gold Medals with their unified softball teams. They also led fund raising efforts such as "Cops and Lobsters" where Tim and other deputies volunteered to wait tables in uniform at the Red Lobster and then donated the earnings to Special Olympics. For several years, Sgt. Thacker led the Olympic Torch Relay through Walton County, a state wide event geared towards generating awareness of Special Olympics and raising funds for the Special Olympics events.

Tim continued to be an awesome father to his children and always attended their activities from cheerleading to marching band, 4H, and tennis. It was a given... Daddy was always there! Tim loved his children deeply and even played "His Majesty" at a reenactment of Cinderella's Ball for his daughters sweet 16 and 14 birthdays. He took his role very seriously... LOL. He played a special song for each of them that night and danced their first slow dance with each of them. It was a tender moment. Tim's office had photos of his wife and daughters proudly displayed.

Everyone who knew Tim Thacker knew he was a man of integrity. A member or the Walton County SWAT Team, he served as a sniper. His accomplishments included becoming a certified firearm and shotgun instructor and a Field Training Officer. He enjoyed his work at the gun range.

Tim found joy in assisting other officers with their shooting techniques and was often quoted as saying "Trigger Control" in their ears as they were firing. He was also an avid re-loader and took pride in recycling shells. He worked his last three years as a criminal investigator in CID, mostly person-to-person crimes. This work weighed heavily on Tim and he often talked of transferring out and returning to the road.

Off duty, Tim loved NASCAR and camping (thanks to his sister-in-law and brother-in-law, Vickie and Danny Hogg). He quickly realized he could sweet talk his way into any race track infield or garage just with his smile and kind words. He took a love for photography, often photographing the drivers before and after the races. Tim even started a small photo business for his daughter, Jocelyn, called "U Name It Photos." Some of their best work included photos for Corralejo's Mexican Grill in Grayson, Georgia. Together, he and Jocelyn carefully shot each plate of deliciously prepared Mexican cuisine for their menu, but most of his photography experience came from shooting crime scenes with his partner, Bo Huff.

Tim enjoyed down time as a brother and proud member of the Masonic Lodge in Loganville and boy could they cook some good Brunswick Stew! Tim grew to enjoy simple pleasures such as watching *Smallville* (the Superman series) and *CSI Las Vegas*, a weekly date for him and his wife. Another popular event in the Thacker household was UFC Fight Night. Tim and Pam would entertain friends with good food, fellowship and laughter. There were many exciting events that happened in 2006 and 2007.

On October 9, 2006, Tim turned the Big "40" and his wife surprised him with a trip to Texas where they attended the OU vs. Texas A&M game in Temple and then stayed in a delightful horse ranch cottage. Tim managed not only to watch the game on the sidelines beside the OU cheerleaders but made friends with several officers there. Texas A&M Sergeant Allan Baron simply walked him out on the field to meet Coach Bob Stoops and as far as Tim Thacker was concerned, life was complete, especially after OU won the game by one point! OU Officer Steve Chandler shared with Tim every reason he should come to Oklahoma and seek employment. They were all so encouraging of Tim's dream.

Tim always wanted to visit Oklahoma and see where he was born. It was a trip his father used to talk of taking with him one day. So, in August of 2007, his wife surprised him for their 20th wedding anniversary with tickets for the whole family to fly to Oklahoma for vacation. They were able to tour the university and before it was over, they were in the president's office. President Boren even invited them to dinner and encouraged them to move and make OU their new home. Pam surprised Tim with two interviews: one with Cleveland County, Oklahoma and the other with the Campus Police at OU. Tim was so very excited! The family enjoyed a delightful time in Oklahoma and Tim pursued employment there.

Before he could make his dream of working for OU come true, he found his work consuming him. After working a very brutal double homicide (with sixty hours of overtime in two weeks), the family found themselves in an unusual predicament. Tim struggled with four weeks of sleep deprivation and a battle of dealing with the images in his mind he simply could not put away. His behavior grew very A-Typical and was followed by several episodes of what the experts call "Triggered events."

Tim Thacker, the husband, the father and friend we knew and loved, was mentally and emotionally overwhelmed. On February 28, 2008, at approximately 9:15 a.m., Tim sent a text to his wife that said "Please forgive me. Thank you for twenty years of wonderful marriage. Thank you for two beautiful girls, please take care of them for me. Things will be better when I'm gone. I have made my peace with God and now I'm going home to meet my maker. Again, please forgive me. You were right about me. You knew me better than I knew myself. Love, Tim." At approximately 9:25 on that same date, Timothy B. Thacker, an American Hero, died at his own hand.

Tim always asked Pam to "push every button" if anything ever happened to him. He would say over and over throughout the years, "You know they don't take care of us in Police work; someone has to help the guys." It appeared in the days following Tim's death, that he had helped everyone but himself, as officer after officer confessed that they too had recently contemplated suicide: yesterday, last week, last month. They related that Tim Thacker had disarmed them or said "That should be me lying in that casket."

It was made apparent through Tim B. Thacker's death that immediate plans for debriefing were necessary and could no longer be optional. Many agencies today still have no protocol for debriefing after a traumatizing scene and officers are left to process what they have witnessed, on their own. Tim had shared with his wife just two days before his death, that he had worked crime scene person to person cases for three years and *never had one day of debriefing*. In Tim's death, many were rescued and several marriages reconciled.

One of Tim's favorite Bible verses: "Greater love has no man than this, that he lay down his life for his friends" (John 15:13, NIV). Sergeant T.B. Thacker was that kind of man. He is dearly missed every single day.

Letter to Timothy Thacker from Pamela F. Thacker (Wife)

Dear Tim,

Thank you for being my high school sweetheart for four years. Thank you for being a supportive husband for 20 years. Thank you for being a wonderful father for 17+ years. Thank you for serving our community through law enforcement for over 18 years. Thank you for being my best friend for 24 years. Thank you for your final text message and your kind words of assurance that you made peace with God and asked him to forgive you. Please take that Masonic Sword Shane gave you and use it to keep Satan away from us and protect us from the evil that we know firsthand is in this world. If you are ever in our presence, I pray you can reveal yourself to us somehow. I pray God allows you to supernaturally comfort our children from above.

Please personally thank God for sending our girls an extra special guardian angel, aka Kevin Brittingham. At the time of your death I don't know what we would've done without him. Please intercede for protection of Robbie and every member of our new blended family.

You would be so proud of our girls. Kristian will graduate this year, a Criminal Justice Major. She has shared her experiences and has helped young soldiers battling PTSD and other students battling with suicidal thoughts. Jocelyn was named Prom Queen and Student of the Year. Our baby is now a Photography Major and you would absolutely love the work she has done. Please help the children to dissolve any feelings they may have that keep them from moving forward and loving life once again. Reveal to us how we can play a vital role in the prevention of

Post Traumatic Stress and helping prevent this destruction from happening to others.

Our fond memories of life and laughter with you, Sgt. T.B. Thacker will forever live on in our hearts. You are always missed and never forgotten—Boomer Sooner!

With you always,
    Pamela F. Thacker

Letter to Tim Thacker from Kristian (Daughter)

Dear Dad,

I miss you. That's a freaking great starter. Let me catch you up with my life. Your oldest daughter is about to graduate from college and just think, I haven't borrowed a dime. I am so impressive. I'm following in your footsteps except I'm going bigger. I start my internship this summer and I'm crossing my fingers the GBI will fall right into place. Dad, Dahlonega is so pretty. You would love it here; right now it's freezing though.

Oh how I want you to see it. My house is wonderful, at first a little overdramatic but things have all worked out even though I need you here to fix some house stuff. And who would have thought, Kristian Thacker, a sorority girl? You wouldn't have, I know that much! I have been in Delta Zeta now for two years and I love it! I have an amazing Little (a "little" is a Sorority Sister) that you always loved, Maggs. Dad, she is amazing. I would have never made it through everything if I didn't have her there by my side. I took her as a little because I can never repay her for the time she spent with me after everything happened. She has grown up so much and misses you as much as everyone else. You would be so proud of everything we are accomplishing together.

I can't even put into words how amazing my life is right now. Not only am I making the right decisions at the right time , but I'm also doing what is best for me and living my life to the fullest. I have had a really hard time putting my wall down in college. I just can't let myself get hurt again by someone I love and I've worked really hard to overcome that. It has pretty much taken a year or so but I'm now back to the person that I was just three years ago. I have gotten to experience so many things since I've been in college. There are so many opportunities I never realized that I could ever have. All my teachers love me, I have been adopted by a couple of families, and I have the ultimate support system... Delta Zeta.

Dad, I have been out of the country! I never thought that was going to happen. Last summer I went to Aruba with the Postma family. They have helped me find joy again. The Postmas are my new family.

I love each and every one of them so very much. They have treated me as if I was part of their own family and always want me around which warms my heart. I only wish I could express to them in words how much I appreciate everything they have done for me over the past year. I first met the Postmas when I started dating Brian. Oh dad, he's the man I'm going to marry! He is everything you ever wanted for me and I'm so glad I listened to you all of those years. Brian wants to meet you so badly! I have told him everything about you, from all those years we spent shooting together to how hilarious you are, not to mention your dashing good looks. Dad, he is taking very, very good care of me. He is everything I have ever wanted in a significant other.

One thing I have been very adamant about is journaling when I am overwhelmed. Dad, I am constantly writing down all the memories. Not because I want to remember, but because I never want to forget. I have established that even three years later, I'm still as hurt and it's a fresh hurt wound. One thing I constantly find myself writing about: is the nagging pain ever going away? And I've answered that question. No, the pain isn't going away. I hurt very badly every morning and night. I can't let go. The one thing I want more than anything is a hug. I just wanted one final hug and a kiss to let me know that everything was going to be okay. You are missing out on everything. I am doing so very well in college, the sorority, and relationship wise. I can't emphasize that enough.

For the longest time I blamed myself. Wondering if it would have made any more of a difference if I just would have texted you back that morning. Then I finally came to the conclusion that it wouldn't have. I would have still ended up in the same place I am currently in today. I also constantly have recurring nightmares about that day. The only thing I ask of you is to make them go away. I can't keep having sleepless nights where I stay up wishing to hear your voice and where I'm too scared to go to sleep.

I need to move on and I feel like there is something you are trying to tell me. I don't understand so, if you could relay that message in a different way, it would be awesome.

I have been trying to write an ending to this letter for about six months now and I have been struggling. I don't want to say goodbye but then again I feel like it is necessary to move on into the next chapter in my life.

Don't worry though, I always think about you and how you need to be here living every chapter of my life with me. You are the best father. I could never ask for anything better than you because no one could have been a better father than you. Thanks for always setting me straight when I was acting a fool, giving me the best advice ever, and raising me to be respectful. Dad, most importantly, thank you for loving me with your whole heart. There is no one who is going to love me as much as you did and no one will ever take your place. You have taught me what it is like to be an absolute fantastic parent. I can't wait to make you proud of all the things I am going to accomplish in life. Whatever you do, never stop believing in me regardless of where life takes me. I need your support too.

I will Love You Forever and Always,

Kristian

Letter to Tim from Jocelyn (Daughter)

Dear Dad,

I miss you like crazy but I know you are looking down at me very proud. I'm now a freshman in college majoring in photography. I have a wonderful boyfriend, roommates, and friends. My boyfriend, Tucker, is really great and I think you would approve of him. He is very nice and treats me great. My roommates are Jessica, Taylor, and Bethany. They're all fun and make me laugh. When I look at your picture, I think of all the great memories we had, especially playing video games together. I remember playing Guitar Hero and you "Rocking Out."

You were such an amazing father. I know that you loved me so very much. I love you so much and always will.

From my situation, I'm able to tell others my story and help them. Things that have happened have made me a better person and taught me to look at life from a different perspective. I want teenagers to be thankful for everything God has provided for them, especially their parents. I will never forget all the things you did for me, how you taught me to make the right decision at the right time, all the time. I love you very much and miss you, but I know you are always watching over me. I was and always will be your Baby Joce.

Romans 5:3-5 (TNIV): "Not only so, but we also glory in our sufferings, because we know that suffering produces perseverance; perseverance, character; and character, hope. And hope does not put us to shame, because God's love has been poured out into our hearts through the Holy Spirit, who has been given to us." (My favorite verse).

Love you Always, Your daughter, Jocelyn J

Letter to Tim from Sabrina Hall Kabay (Friend)

Dear Tim,

Thank you for always being there for me. Like a big brother to the rescue when I needed it! I can see you now, walking up our driveway for the first time to welcome my family to the neighborhood. You were in your "camos," boots, and beret, with your dog, Rambo, by your side (you were the only one to welcome us by the way).

You always marched to a different beat, and stood out more than others, but in a good way! The world was a much better place with you in it! You had a heart of gold, and a beautiful soul!

I can't wait to see you again my friend.

Some day, Sabrina Hall Kabay

Letter to Tim from Em (Friend)

To Mr. Thacker... aka Tim... aka Fruitcake:

I really don't know where to begin. I guess I would start with saying that when I think about how your earthly life ended and the pain you must've felt, I hurt. When I found out that you were gone, my heart broke and I knew I had lost a friend who had been dying inside. You had to have been hurting. I say this without a doubt because the Tim that I knew would have fought anyone or anything who tried to take his life away (or anyone else's life for that matter).

You loved life. You adored your wife and your children. You loved God and being a positive role model to young children. You spent most of your time protecting and influencing other lives by choice. I feel special to have been one of those teens who really got to know the real Tim Thacker. I think about how you would appear to be such a rough and indestructible guy, but then when you dug into who you were personally, it was clear that you were just a big softy. Your life is reassurance that counseling is vital in the lives of everyone. I plan on taking that passion I possess and helping beautiful people like you.

I want to say "Thank You" for the times you have helped me. Growing up in church, you were along for the ride, being my Sunday School Teacher and supervising on trips. In looking back, I know how important my down time is as an adult and it probably took a lot for you to volunteer and be around crazy teens. We had a lot of fun though. You would never put on that 'Big Bad Tim' front with me, because you knew that I knew you were deeper than that. I am sure that was because you were nurturing two girls who were pre-teens. I know that you truly cared about me and the rest of the group. Through time, a role model evolved into a friend as well.

Even after I graduated from high school, we ran into each other and you would make sure to let me know that you remembered the good times. Time with me and the group was meaningful to you. You reminded me of the person that I am. I was always thrilled to see you because you knew the real me. In fact, the last time I saw you, you helped with a situation that I was very concerned about. You reassured me that I would be protected and I walked out without a fear. When you said something, you meant it. Thank you for protecting all of us through your faithful service.

I am sure that you know how much you are thought of, loved and missed. I wonder what you guys are doing there in heaven. Are you chillin' with my Uncle Hugh? I know God has a plan for everything, but this is so hard to understand when those who are so special leave so soon. Know that your story has had no ending. It is being used to better the world. I pray that one day soon, counseling will be seen as a necessary outreach for everyone. Life is hard.

Even the tough fall hard and when this happens, it's a lot easier to get up when there is a "springboard." I love you, Fruitcake. Your soul is at rest. Watch over us and enjoy your heaven.

Your friend,
     Em

Letter to Tim from Jeff (Cousin)

Dear Tim,

Writing you this letter is the hardest thing I have had to do because you are gone now. I can't put into words how much I miss you other than by saying my life will never be the same without you. Since your passing, my life has finally turned around for the better and there are so many wonderful things I wish I could tell you about, for instance: the fact that I live in Loganville now and that both of my children are on their way to college. I have finally found a good job and am able to make a good living and have even been able to purchase a new truck. Although it's not a Chevrolet, I know you would still be very happy for me.

You used to tell me "Keep your chin up Bodine, good things are going to come your way" and you were right because I have found the most wonderful woman in the world and I married her. The only thing that is missing is my cousin Tim, aka Torrell, and the fact that I can't share all this wonderful news and the great happenings in my life with you. Even though we promised each other when we became old men and retired, we would sit on the front porch in rocking chairs and gripe about politics while our grandchildren played in the yard, now that you are gone, no one will ever be able to fill that void. You were always like the brother I never had.

I loved you and miss you with all my heart. Whenever I drive past the cemetery where you are buried and see your beautiful marker, it is no comparison to the person you were and the impact you had on my life. You knew everything about me and whenever you told me I was in the wrong, I listened. Other than the grandparents we shared, your wisdom and advice and your love meant everything to me.

As long as I live, I will never forget you and whenever I reminisce about the times we had together, all I can do is smile and laugh and feel warm inside because we had nothing but good times together as cousins, parents, and friends. I loved you with all my heart and the hardest thing I ever had to do was say goodbye.

With all my heart, Your cousin Jeff aka Bodine

Letter to Tim From Melanie Cooksey (Professional Contact)

Dear Tim,

I remember the day I met you at the Sheriff's Office in Monroe in April, 2007. I was being harassed from 3000 miles away by my ex-husband's new wife for no reason. I came to you two years after it started and it had escalated to involve my job and the people I work with.

I brought all of the evidence I had saved over the previous two years along with all the new evidence that was currently going on at that time. I really didn't know what to expect, but after talking with you, you decided to take my statement and begin a long distance investigation into this woman who lived on the west coast. You taught me how to look up the IP addresses to the emails I had begun receiving from a person I didn't know and how that IP address would tell us where the computer was that it was coming from. It was then that we were able to get hard evidence against this girl on the west coast.

I will never forget, from the months of April, 2007 through October, 2007, the conversations we had about my case and you always apologizing for not getting back to me as promptly as you liked, due to several other horrific cases you were working on that involved children. Even with your more pressing and important cases, you still spent the time needed on my case and took it before the Grand Jury.

I received the best birthday gift I could ever receive on my birthday October 26, 2007. You called me that day to let me know the Grand Jury had just indicted this girl on four Felony Counts and eight Misdemeanors and that she would have to fly to Georgia to appear in court due to the Felonies involved. It wasn't until February, 2008, at her first court appearance, that I had the opportunity to see and speak with you again. It was clear that she was going to be convicted on all charges and would now be a convicted felon.

My family came in support and I remember seeing you walk in and pointing you out to them as I said "My hero, the person who didn't think my case was insignificant and pursued an arrest." I made sure before we parted ways that day, that I approached you and thanked you for all of your hard work and support on this case. It was because of you that there was a conviction and that she is currently serving five years probation as a convicted felon with the possibility of 48 years in prison if she violates her First Offender status.

I wanted to be sure you knew how thankful I was to you.

I am so glad I took that opportunity to let you know because just a day later, I learned you had committed suicide due to Post Traumatic Stress. It broke my heart, but at the same time, I was so happy that you knew how thankful I was. I will always be grateful for your help and will never forget you.

Sincerely,
Melanie Cooksey

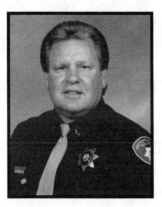

CHRISTOPHER VAN CLEEF
December 28, 1957—September 30, 2008
Biography by Joyce Van Cleef (Wife)

Christopher Joseph Van Cleef, the son of William and Marie Van Cleef was born in Brooklyn, New York on a cold winter's day, December 28, 1957. Chris' family moved to Las Vegas, Nevada when he was a child. Chris graduated from Clark High School, one of the oldest high schools in Las Vegas, in 1975.

Chris stayed in Vegas after high school and at the young age of 22, he was hired as a police officer with the Las Vegas Metropolitan Police Department. Law Enforcement however, was not his only passion. Chris was an avid musician and he absolutely loved music. In his early years he was in a fantastic band named "Red Bush." Also in the band were his best friends, Bob Buettner and Gary Higby. Influenced by the Beatles, the Eagles, and Fleetwood Mac, they played classic rock songs about love and togetherness. Chris played in the band until his obligations as a father and a police officer became too demanding for him to juggle all three roles. He did play with a band regularly though as he got older, that band was comprised of Chris himself and his boys and they jammed in the music room at home all of the time.

They were able to do so because that same love Chris had for music was passed on to his boys.

Chris was married to Joyce for nearly his entire adult life and they had three boys together: Justin, Sean, and Cory. Chris and Joyce lived with every breath their children took. Chris was like many others and loved sports, holidays and good movies. His favorite football team was the Pittsburgh Steelers and his favorite holiday was Christmas. Chris often said the two best seasons of the year were Christmas Season and Football Season. His favorite colors were even Black and Gold (go figure).

Chris' hobbies included gardening and putting out bird feeders to attract Humming Birds. This is kind of funny because had you seen Chris, you most likely would have described him as many others did. He was a tough looking cop and was built solid like a fire plug (as many would say). He was intimidating to many people but he was gentle to the core of his heart. In addition to Humming Birds and flowers, Chris loved visiting his family's favorite vacation spot... their cabin in Cedar City, Utah. When there, Chris spent most of his time hanging with the family, fishing, riding ATVs and relaxing with everyone (friends and family) by the fire. Chris truly enjoyed a good movie. He liked dramas to comedies.

Of the many movies he loved, *Tombstone* and *Unforgiven* were his favorites along with anything with Chris Farley in it. He also loved television and would often watch classics like *Bonanza* and *M*A*S*H*, along with more recent shows like *The King of Queens*.

A dedicated police officer, Chris began his career in Patrol (like most other officers) and before he retired more than 25 years later, he had worked in the Narcotics Bureau, Patrol, and he ran the Special Events section of the Las Vegas Metropolitan Police Department which is the unit that handles the issuance of permits and staffing for the filming of movies, commercials, road work, and concerts, to name a few activities. In fact, Chris had denied a permit for one very famous Rock and Roll Band after they had nearly incited a riot the year before. The drummer for the band was so angry, he called and left a voice message on

Chris' answering machine at work and called him every name in the dictionary and then some. Part of being a cop as Chris put it. He progressed through the police levels all the way to the rank of Lieutenant.

Most importantly, Chris Van Cleef was a caring person who put nearly everyone before himself and would often help people who had abused his kindness multiple times. He was an extraordinary man who touched all who knew him.

Chris Van Cleef, an American Hero, took his own life in Henderson, Nevada on September 30, 2008.

Letter to Chris from Joyce (Wife)

My Dearest Chris,

It has been a little over two years since you left us and I can't even put into words how much I miss you. You were the love of my life and my best friend since I was 14. When you first left, I was so mad at you. How could you have left us without giving us a chance to talk to you? You had no right to make that decision for me. Now I am left all alone without my best friend and your boys don't have the father they loved so much.

Remember when they were little and you would get down on the floor and wrestle with them? Until they got so big you said "I can't do this anymore because I can't see the third one coming." You were such a wonderful dad and it makes me so sad that our grandchildren are never going to get to know their grandfather. You would have been such a good grandpa.

I still can't believe that you are never going to be part of our lives anymore. We grew up together and I always took for granted that we were going to grow old together. It is true what they say "Don't ever take anything for granted." Chris, you were such a good person, you would do anything for anyone, even if it caused you hardship. You stood for what you thought was right no matter who got mad.

I will never forget your sense of humor and the silly things you made me do like pretend we were asleep when you saw the boys walk up the pathway to the house when they came home from school. You gave so much to our boys, your love of music was something wonderful. The song you wrote for me, I will cherish forever. Your sons are sweet and caring people just like their dad and I will make sure they stay that way. When they have families, I will make sure your grandchildren will know what a wonderful person their grandpa was.

I just want you to know that I know you were hurting a lot inside and that I am not mad at you. I also hope that you are not sad anymore and you are at peace. Hopefully, if it's true what they say, we will be together again and I am going to hug you so hard that you will never leave me again. I love you and miss you so very much my heart feels like it is torn in half, but I feel so lucky for the time that I did have with you. I will cherish those memories forever.

I love you,
Joyce (Kiddo)

Letter to Chris from Sean (Son)

"Look around you. Everything you see, I own." Dad, when you used to say those few sentences, they were meant to be a funny reminder to us who the sheriff in town was at our house whenever we got out of line or didn't want to do our chores. I had no idea, until you were gone, that it meant much more than that. Just by the number of people who showed up to your memorial service, it could be seen that you owned a special place in each one of their hearts. No one's attention diverted from the stage as friends and family came up to share special moments, heartfelt and funny ones.

As a dad, you could make me laugh when we would poke fun of our relatives at family gatherings, anger me to no end whenever you had to bring down the iron fist of parental justice, annoy me with constant requests for me to imitate Austin Powers because of that one time I did it, and keep me company when we would watch Bonanza or Escape from New York. You were always there for me, and you are one of the biggest influences on the person that I've come to be.

And, above all else, what made you such a great father, and human being in general, was your constant support of myself, Justin and Cory, while still guiding us along so we planned for the future.

No matter if it was playing in bands, or supporting us as we went through High School and College, you never stopped being a great dad, even though you were constantly stressed out from working with the police department.

Dad, I love you, and if we ever do get to see each other one last time, as much as it will pain me to do so, I know what my first words to you will be. "Yeah, baby!"

Letter to Chris from Justin (Son)

Dear dad,

It's been awhile since I last saw you, almost two and a half years now. Whereas I don't get as emotional as a couple years ago when I remember you, I still miss you incredibly. You really were the keystone in my life, alongside mom. Everything I have and who I have become is in direct correlation with the nature of my upbringing.

Day to day, some event will come up that reminds me of you, whether it be a football game, a great western movie, or simply, a tasty beer. I often wonder what input you'd have on some of the traveling I have done since you passed, as well as how much the stories would make you smile. Man, I miss your sense of humor. Luckily, I still experience it slightly in Sean and Cory.

Although things are better now, I still really wish you had rethought the decision you made that cold, September morning. I know that you were going through a lot, however, I thought you were allowing me to help you through it. Was asking for help really that hard? Was it worth not getting to see the careers your sons would find or the grandchildren you'd help raise? I know you weren't in a normal state of mind when it happened but I still sincerely wish you would have held out longer to gather your senses and realize what you were leaving behind.

You can't hear these words now, but you still are the reason I am educated enough to write them. You were one fantastic father and an overall amazing human being who would do anything for your wife and sons, and for that, I thank you. We all still miss you more that grammatically possible to explain, and I don't ever see that changing. I love you dad.

Love, Justin

Letter to Chris from Christopher Cory (Son)

Dad,

I don't know where to begin this letter considering I have so much that I wish I could say to you. I suppose I'll start with the day you left us because I remember it more than I'd like to , but what I remember most is what you said to me before I went to school. You told me that everything was going to be okay and then you gave me a hug like I've never had before and probably won't have ever again. Later on when you told me to take care of mom and to go be with her, I knew what was happening.

I'm so mad at you for lying to me, dad. Nothing was okay. You left your family to figure out what the hell was going on when none of us had any idea what to do. And I'm most angry at you for leaving mom the way you did. She did not deserve any of this and seeing what your absence did to her at the beginning was absolutely horrendous. The fact that there was nothing that Justin, Sean or I could articulate to her to make her feel any better still leaves me feeling vacant. You should have realized that you didn't need to do what you did. We just needed you and still do.

What takes away the angst I feel for the situation is how much I love you. I love how much you still shine in all of our lives and how not a single hour goes by that I don't think of you or what you would do in my situation. It's funny how the most minute experiences or feeling can bring you to mind.

I still can't hear an Eagles song without thinking about you and I can't listen to a single Redbush song without crying. It just reminds me how much I want to talk to you. How much I want to tell you about what's going on in my life and hopefully have you feel proud of me. Every time something happens in my life that I'm pleased with, the first thought that comes to mind is how you'll never know.

It can make being proud a little less exciting sometimes.

And even though I completely disagree with your final decision, I still look up to you. You and mom are the two greatest, most selfless people I've ever had the luck to be around. When we were growing up, every choice was in favor of us kids and every experience that was given, shaped me to be who I am today. I can't thank you enough for teaching me to enjoy and appreciate what I have and not to take it for granted. You and mom really showed me what is important to hold on to.

If I could relive any point in my life, I know exactly which time it would be. The summer that the cabin was being built would be my choice, hands down. You and I drove up almost every week to check on the progress and once it was possible to stay in it, you were so excited. But those drives to Utah are my favorite part. Talking about music and telling each other about our favorite concept album, dissecting our favorite parts to each other. Or listening to talk radio and laughing at how ridiculous some of the subject matter was. I also remember you letting me drive the Excursion on the highway for the first time. I was so terrified I had to pull over and you teased me about it the rest of the way home. That still brings a smile to my face.

I can't believe how long it's been already. From the moment you left us, every day was so bleak and it was so hard to get back into normal life, if that is even what I'd call it now that we don't have you anymore. I wish I could tell you how much we miss you. I wish we could just have you back. But instead, I'll just say that we love you so much. I love you so much, dad. I miss you as a father, but I mainly miss you as my friend.

Love, Christopher Cory

Letter to Chris from Vicki (Sister)

Dear Chris,

I do not think I can put into writing how much I miss you. I think about you every day, especially when I see a hummingbird, watch the Steelers (Yes, I really do watch the Steelers and Heinz Ward is so cute on Dancing with the Stars), eat pizza and wings or listen to the m at night to take care of herusic that we both love. I wish you had let me know what you were going through. I might have been able to help but I guess we'll never know if that was possible.

When you were little you were so cute. You reminded me of a little penguin. When I had Jen, you stayed up late at night to take care of her when I had to work. You took care of everyone else's kids. You should be here for your boys and grandchildren.

Nothing will ever be the same. In the time that has passed I have gotten closer to Joyce but further from everyone else. When you left us, I knew that the glue that kept our family together was gone too. I feel cheated without you but you cheated yourself more.

You won't get to attend all of the special events in your son's futures or spend the vacations with Joyce, John, and I that we talked about in our later years. The night before you died you asked me to stand by Joyce's side. I only wish that you were standing next to us!

Your loving sister and friend, Vicki

P.S. "You'll be in my heart" and always on my speed dial
for our late night talks

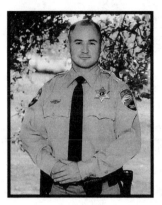

MATTHEW ZIELINSKI
February 4, 1978—June 1, 2005
Biography by Julie Zielinski (Mother)

Matthew was the middle child in the Zielinski family with an older sister, Tami, and a younger brother, Mark. He grew up in Wenatchee, Washington, where his extended family included numerous cousins, aunts, and uncles, as well as beloved grandparents.

His parents are both teachers and tennis coaches, so sports were a huge part of Matthew's life. Soccer and baseball were favorites in elementary school, and he played tennis throughout his life.

In the winter season, Matthew played hockey from age five until his death. The first year as a player, he didn't really know how to skate. He would hit the puck and fall down, get up and repeat it all over again. He finally became a good skater, scoring many hat tricks, playmakers, and lots of assists.

He always wanted to sit in the penalty box. The first time he received a penalty, he had the biggest grin on his face. He'd finish his time, spot another innocent victim and take off after that person. Finally, his mother explained that his penalties were hurting his team. That still didn't stop his aggressiveness. In high school he earned several "Most Improved Player" awards and was an asset to his team. While he also played middle school and high school football, hockey remained his favorite sport. He was the poster boy for the Bible verse, "Whatever your hand finds to do, do it with all your might" (Ecclesiastes 9:10, NIV).

In August 1987, when Matthew was entering fourth grade,

his grandparents took the family to Honolulu, staying at the Hale Koa for a week. His Grandfather S. showed the family around the military base where he was stationed during WWII, and they ate lunch together at one of his grandfather's favorite spots. Grandpa S. also showed them the historical sites honoring the USS Arizona and Pearl Harbor. Maybe that is where the idea took root in Matthew to become a United States Marine.

One day toward the end of his junior year in high school, Matthew talked to the Marine Corps recruiters who were visiting the school. He immediately wanted to become a Marine. Because he was not yet 18, his parents had to sign for him at the recruiting office, a day of high excitement for Matthew. Grandfather S. would have been thrilled, since he had been a Lieutenant Commander in the Navy.

Matt worked hard at keeping in shape and meeting with the recruiters through his senior year. He graduated on a Friday, had a farewell party on Saturday, and he was off to boot camp on Sunday, June 9, 1996. Weeks later, graduation day arrived, and part of his family went to the Marine Corps Recruit Depot near San Diego, California for the ceremony. The drill sergeants gave a brief talk, followed by a dinner. The recruits marched over.

Matt was in Company 2122: upright posture, standing tall and proud in his perfectly pressed uniform. The impeccably dressed young man gave his mother a big hug and talked briefly. Matt was now a self-assured and self-confident leader.

He was first assigned to Camp Pendleton for further training, and then to Chesapeake, Virginia to serve on the Security Force Battalion. At some point, he was stationed at Bangor Naval Base in the state of Washington, about four hours west of Wenatchee. He was then sent to Bahrain on the USS Nimitz, Marine Detachment, assigned to the search for terrorists. In 1998, after being overseas and serving on the USS Nimitz, he headed to Yorktown, Virginia. In 1999 Matthew was promoted to Sergeant.

By April, he was stationed in Japan, but his captain agreed to allow him leave to join his family in Hawaii for a family reunion. Matthew arrived before the rest of the family (26 in all) and was waiting for them. When Grandpa Z's and Matthew's eyes met, it was an indescribable picture of love and respect. The family stayed at the Aston Kaanapali Shores, enjoying special times on the beautiful grounds and at the pool. The boy cousins played tennis and, as usual, Matthew won. The days also included beach time, a visit to Lahaina Park, and lunch with the immediate family. Matthew had matured and changed, but he still loved being with and playing with the little cousins. At the airport, his huge smile faded and a frown appeared, as he left his family to return to duty.

In 2000, Matthew was home after four years in the Marines. Sister Tami, her husband, Brad, and Matthew's three-month-old niece, Alexis, were visiting in Wenatchee. Tami loved waking up her brother because it always made him so mad. But, this time was different—he was meeting Alexis for the very first time. With eyes half open, a smile crossed his face and he held her for the first time. He loved kids and he looked so natural holding his adorable little Lexi.

Matthew decided to attend Whatcom Community College in Bellingham, Washington to earn his Associates Degree. He had to complete two years of college in order to become a Sheriff's Deputy. He had plans to get a four year degree at Washington State University at some point during his career as a deputy. While attending college, he worked at Skagit Valley

Casino as a security officer. At the end of the school year, Matthew moved back to Wenatchee to finish his degree at Wenatchee Valley College.

At some point during these years, Matt became a Christian. Even though he had attended church all his life, he had finally asked Jesus into his heart.

While he intensely longed to rejoin the military and head to the war in Iraq, the pull of his dream of working in law enforcement in central Washington won his heart. In July, 2004, the Chelan County Sheriff's Office hired him as a deputy. Within two weeks he was in Spokane, Washington at the Washington State Basic Law Enforcement Academy, Session 574. Matthew graduated from the Academy on December 1, 2004.

His brother and mother attended the graduation ceremony, along with representatives of the Chelan County Sheriff's Office. After the events of the day were over, the Sheriff told Matthew he had two days off and then he would be starting work. He could hardly wait.

His duty began by training with the Field Training Officers (FTOs) for fourteen weeks. Even though he knew what was expected of him as a deputy, he was afraid he wouldn't make the cut with the FTOs. One of the officers he trained with said that he was a good deputy. Matt knew that he was being assigned to the SWAT Team effective July 1, an unusual assignment for a new deputy. Usually there is a two year wait to be on the SWAT Team, but because of his extensive military training, they made an exception. In the meantime, his assignment was to the night shift around Lake Chelan.

Matthew really cared about people. In his resume, written as part of his application to the Sheriff's Office, that was one quality that stood out. He didn't really want to arrest people, he wanted to help them turn their lives around. He was a very kind young man, with a soft heart, but he could be tough when he had to be.

Matthew John Zielinski, an American hero, died at his own hand on June 1, 2005.

The following are some of the statements made at Matt's Funeral Service:

> Matthew's life-long dream of becoming a Deputy Sheriff with Chelan County came true on July 1, 2004. Matthew continued his service to our country as a Deputy Sheriff for Chelan County. He stated in his application for employment with the Sheriff's Office, "I have a sincere desire to contribute to law enforcement efforts within Chelan County. I enjoy helping others with their problems." Although a quiet person, Matthew's true dedication to helping others showed every day he put on his uniform, stepped into his patrol car, and said, "K63 in service."

> One of the first times I met Matt was on a SWAT training day, and we needed a role player to assist us in the training exercise. I was impressed with Matt's quiet demeanor, high and tight haircut, his sense of commitment, duty, honor, and his experience in the Marine Corps as a Fast Company Member. Their mission was both a Counter Terrorist Mission and a Security Mission, protecting Special Nuclear Materials on board ships, and in port.

On the one hand, he was the tough law enforcement officer. But beneath the harsh exterior, lay a heart of gold. We may also be comforted in knowing that he was a man of faith. Although he did not express it in conventional ways, Matthew put his faith in God.

So, in the midst of our sadness, in the middle of our unending questions of "Why?" we may find comfort in knowing that Matthew, the Marine Sergeant, who became a Chelan County Sheriff's Deputy, has now left for a new assignment. His new beat is heaven, and he is serving in the Lord's Army!

Letter to Matthew from Julie Zielinski (Mother)

Dear Matthew,

As I write you this letter it has been 5 years, 3 months and 25 days since that tragic phone call at 1:04 in the morning. Your dad and I were in such a state of shock that you would take your own life. We were in shock and disbelief. They told us everything and they were so sincere and caring at the loss of one of their own— Deputy Matthew Zielinski.

The only reason I am here today is because God has held me up. You were such a good looking, tough, yet compassionate young man with a huge heart. You were a great athlete and I loved watching you grow from a five year old hockey player who fell down every time you hit the puck to a good hockey player scoring and assisting your team to victory throughout high school. We often talk of all your funny ways, usually at the dinner table. You always made me laugh even though I should have been punishing you for something you did that was not appropriate. Often I hear you say something like "Don't drive my Yukon!" You took great pride in that vehicle and you didn't want anyone to drive it. Well, you left, so now I am driving your vehicle.

I was so proud of you when you became a United States Marine. I asked you once why you wanted to be a Marine when you didn't like people telling you what to do. You said, "Why do you think I moved up in rank so fast? So I could be in charge of my men!" And then, after your time in the Marines was up, you finished your education and landed your dream career as a Chelan County Sheriff Deputy. You were so handsome in both uniforms. You truly grew into a wonderful young man. I loved when you would call me and tell me of a traffic stop or an arrest. You knew I loved action and you never failed to keep me informed.

We were very close and you knew you could come to me for anything. I just wish you had called me that night. I would have been there in a second to try to save you. I always supported you in all that you did.

My heart is broken in a million pieces and I will never be the same again. As I write my book about your life: *A Life Too Short: Matt's Story*, I sit in your bedroom surrounded by your Marine and Deputy Sheriff memorabilia. Knowing your heart, I feel like I now understand why you took your own life. However, there was a better way than that. All you needed to do was call me anytime—day or night. As your dad told you when you entered the Marines, "If you ever get in trouble, pray to God. He is the only One who can help you." I feel you didn't want the embarrassment of being rejected. I figure if you had one more second, you would not have done what you did.

I can only move on with my life knowing you are with God. Through his love I will be okay. I miss you every moment of my life. All I can do is look at your picture daily, talk to you and visit your grave site weekly, if not more often. You made me a proud mother with your many accomplishments and I will love you forever. Until we meet in heaven... I will be strong for you.

Love forever and forever,
Mom

CHAPTER 5

WHAT HAPPENS TO A MOTHER'S LITTLE BOY
by Don Webb

The following poem was written by Don Webb, a police officer in North Carolina. Don did not commit suicide nor was he suicidal. However, this poem, *What Happens to a Mother's Little Boy*, describes how thousands of law enforcement officers feel about themselves, their profession, and life, after serving their community for many years.

What Happens to a Mother's Little Boy ?
By Don Webb

What happens to a mother's little boy
As he grows up, and leaves home
To launch his own crusade and struggle
Against evil.

What happens to a Mother's little boy
When he sheds his youth
And enters the world of the aged
When he turns in his cape and boots, for a badge and a gun.

What happens to a Mother's little boy
When he discovers the dark side of humankind
The fear, the hatred, and the ignorance
And the apathy.

What happens to a Mother's little boy
When he cannot reason with a thief
When he cannot convince a victim
When he cannot enlighten a judge
When he cannot sober an addict
When he cannot help the helpless; a child.

What happens to a Mother's little boy
When he is ridiculed by the very people he has sworn to protect
What happens when he is called a racist,
a failure, an incompetent
A Nazi.

What happens to a Mother's little boy
When he has done all he can, more than most,
And the people say, "You didn't do enough!"
"You should have done more!"

What happens to a Mother's little boy
When the people blame him
"You should have protected us! You should have known
That disturbed and lonely person was a serial killer!"
"That's what you're supposed to do!"

What happens to a Mother's little boy
When the mental patient, who didn't get the help he needed
Targets a school
"You should have helped that poor boy!"
"This is your fault!"

What happens to a Mother's little boy
When the court does not support his actions
And the criminal is set free to
Destroy more lives.
What happens to a Mother's little boy
When he's hit by a drunk driver
And never fully recovers
From the shock and the trauma.

What happens to a Mother's little boy
When the patient cannot be saved
And the bleeding cannot be stopped

When the Sergeant yells, "Forget the first aid kit!
Get the crime scene tape!"
And he stops CPR as the man on the street stares at him
With confused pain and desperate necessity
And then stares at nothing.

What happens to a Mother's little boy
When his department lets him down
"I'm sorry son, you did what I would have done,
But you're on your own."

What happens to a Mother's little boy
When his child wakes up screaming
In the middle of the night, "I had a dream you got hurt!
Please don't go to work tonight, Daddy!"

What happens to a mother's little boy
When his pay, when compared to the hours he works,
Is less than minimum wage
And he can't pay his bills.

What happens to a Mother's little boy
When his wife doesn't understand and he can't explain it
When he's expected to leave work at work
And come home the young man he once was

What happens to a Mother's little boy
When his partner is shot
And he escapes death by an inch,
Or by fate, or by luck, or by cowardice.
What happens to a Mother's little boy
When exhaustion overtakes him
When he can barely move
And when he runs out of answers.
The little boy's spirit breaks
He eats his meals alone
And he sleeps in a cold room by himself.

The little boy tries more than anything
To help others
While he searches for a lost hope.
The more he tries, the more failure he sees...
The little boy sees his little boy fade away
He sees his wife leave him behind
And take everything.

The little boy loses himself
In his crusade
Because he has lost.
The little boy shuns joy; for he does not deserve it
He isolates friends, for he is the only one who failed
He hides his depression as to not appear weak.

He drinks
He eats
He exercises
But in it all
He cries in the
Deepest of despair.
He lives off crumbs, and $200 a month
As his Ex-Family gets the rest
While his body and mind suffer from malnutrition.

As time goes on...
The little boy rejects humanity, as they are not worth saving
He rejects God, as no higher power would allow evil to win
Finally, the little boy rejects himself:
He was a fool to think he could help
He was despised by his citizenry
He has lost everything, for all of them.

The little boy
In one last spasm of shame
Remembers his Mother.
He thinks of his childhood...
Playing outside after school in the mountain air
Eating every meal at the table with everyone else
The warm brick house heated by the wood in the fireplace
The wood he helped chop...
And the worst thought of all enters his distraught mind
"I failed my Mother.
How could I have done such a thing?"
The little boy cannot bear this burden...

What happens to this Mother's little boy?
Will she bury him? Will she take the folded
Flag and never understand what happened to the
Greatest thing that ever happened to her?
Will his child ever know what he tried so
Desperately to do, and that he did it to make the world
Better for her.

Will you thank this little boy?
Will you remember him, or let his efforts
Of which you were unwilling to undertake
Go for naught?
Will you help this little boy
As unselfishly as he tried to help
All of us?
What happens to a Mother's little boy?

CONCLUSION

Writing this book became a far more daunting task than I had anticipated a short four years ago. I thought I would simply put my experiences down on paper and then collect a few biographies for inclusion in the book. I had no idea of the emotional toll *My Life For Your Life* would have on me. Writing my portion of the book, "Cop Stew," wasn't too trying as I tell that same story at every seminar. There are however, nearly always, at least some raw emotions that rise to the surface when I explain the issues that nearly took me down, but time and professional help have brought me back to where I need to be psychologically, and in my life.

As I wrote this book, I realized that Tracie's contribution, "A Day In The Pool," was every bit as necessary as my chapter was. Just as the attendees at our seminars hear the full story, readers of *My Life For Your Life*, needed to read the full story as well. With my introductory chapter, Tracie's contribution, and a clear explanation of Posttraumatic Stress Disorder and Cumulative Stress, written by the respected psychologist, David Joseph, I mistakenly assumed the most difficult portion of creating this book was behind me.

My opinion that the difficult part was complete quickly came to a screeching halt when I spoke with Charlotte Banish, the mother of the late Lieutenant Joseph Banish. Joe was the first officer whose biography was to be included in this book. I truly thought that I would simply collect the biographies, photographs, and letters and place them in order in the book. I never even considered the emotional bond that might develop with some of these family members and friends of these incredible officers. I certainly did not initially feel as if these featured officers were my friends, but upon completion, I felt like they were actually family. I spoke with families via telephone and exchanged emails. Some of the featured officers' family and friends even attended our seminars. A bond with every contributing person and their loved one, the officers, had been cultivated.

I spoke with mothers and fathers. I spoke with sisters, wives and fiancés. Every time I spoke with them via telephone, I had to try to hide the fact that their stories were tearing me apart inside.

Every officer's (and family's) story was heart wrenching and they all carried me on an emotional roller coaster ride. I tried to imagine one of my children taking his or her own life and that thought was absolutely unbearable. I didn't know how any of these incredible people could ever bring themselves to smile again. My pain, insignificant when compared to that of these survivors, I'm sure, did not end there. I still had a book to write. I had to give guidance to all of those contributing. I read every biography and every letter and then, I read them again. Once more I dealt with emotions that I had not anticipated. I eventually learned that before I would read a biography or a letter, I needed to have a box of tissues nearby.

As I read each contribution, it bothered me more and more that these officers did not seek help. In some cases, psychological help was available and the officers not only failed to seek that help, they didn't even accept it when offered. Perhaps some of them weren't even aware of the help available to them. (We will never know.) I'm nearly certain they didn't think that the psychological help, whether provided by a doctor, counselor, or a friend, would even work. Tragically, they were wrong in avoiding the assistance of others. And the great irony is that each of them would be the very first to offer *others* whatever assistance they needed.

I am not a psychologist, nor am I a counselor. I am merely a man who worked as a police officer for most of his adult life (26 years and counting) and spent most of that quarter century socializing with police officer friends. As I noted in "Cop Stew," I never thought police related stress would be a factor in my life. In fact, most new police officers don't think stress is going to be a significant factor in their lives. Unfortunately, as nearly any expert will tell you, stress will most likely play a major role in the lives of virtually every man or woman who wears the police badge. Just as with the officers whose stories are told here, stress will probably be one of the greatest factors in their professional lives.

Only after working with all of the survivors and writing this book did I realize the true importance of educating officers, and everyone in America for that matter, on the hidden dangers of police suicide. *My Life For Your Life* has changed me forever. It changed me as a cop but more importantly as a human being. Stress, PTSD, Depression, and Cumulative Stress can all be dealt with and managed if we only accept the help and guidance available. They can be beaten if we accept help, rather than trying to rely on our own resources alone. They can be managed and it is possible for veteran police officers, upon conclusion of their careers, to feel the same enthusiasm for their jobs as they did when they were rookies.

There are thousands of police officers who struggle every day with the stressors we have addressed in this book and no one can tell which of those officers will accept help, but what we do know is the ones who do seek help, have a far greater chance of living a long, happy and healthy life than those who do not. A life in which they will continue to learn, live, and love. A life in which they will continue to enjoy friends and family and their career. A life in which they can finish out their career and retire and then enjoy a pension and all the experience, memories and satisfaction that comes from serving their communities as one of America's Heroes. And when they do admit their human limits, I can assure you one thing they will say for the rest of that happy life will be, "I am so glad I sought and accepted help!"

Without fear there can be no courage. Should you need help, step up and do for yourself what you would not think twice about doing for others—save a life and get help, so that your loved ones will never have to suffer like these survivors of police suicide. They have willingly shared their own profound grief in the hope that their words just may make a difference in helping you to choose life.

ACKNOWLEDGEMENTS

As any author will tell you, no one writes a book alone. *My Life For Your Life* was no exception. This book would not have been possible without the patience, time, and compassion of not only my wife, Tracie, but our loving children as well. Jessica, Justin, Cristina, Nicolas, Brandon and even my son-in-law Joey, have visited, talked with, and even watched movies as a family while, many times, I sat at the computer working on this book. There were so many times when we would go to dinner as a family and I would bring up *My Life For Your Life*. No one ever complained. (I don't think I could have been that understanding had someone else been so consumed by any single subject.)

The family and friends of the heroes featured in this book were amazing. To lose a loved one to suicide is always one of the worst moments in someone's life and the pain lasts forever. As I read their contributions to this book, I would think to myself how difficult it must have been for them to pen those words. I am thankful to all who contributed, not only family members but friends as well. I hope that participating in this project has helped to bring some healing closure into their lives.

My hope is not only that these great heroes are memorialized, but also that this modest book helps other officers, civilians and military personnel to better understand PTSD, Cumulative Stress and Depression. I hope this book aids law enforcement officers and military personnel who might be struggling, and convinces them that the help that is already in place does work. My thanks and acknowledgements are to those listed above and to all of our nation's heroes and all who work towards saving the lives of those heroes. America has always been a proud nation comprised of noble people. Thank you to everyone who has made it great through their labor, sacrifices, and contributions on behalf of our heroes. Thank you to all who stand ready to help those who on a daily basis risk their own lives so that ours may be protected.

RESOURCES AVAILABLE
TO STRUGGLING OFFICERS

- SafeCallNow.org

- CopsAlive.com

- Employee Assistance Programs

- Peer Support Programs

- Psychologist / Psychiatrist

- Counselors

- Police Chaplains

- Addiction Centers

- Group Therapy

- Church

- Hotlines

- Self Help Groups

- Financial Centers